# PLANT-BASED,

## VEGETARIAN, AND VEGAN DIETS FOR BEGINNERS

The Guide To Improving Your Health And

Saving The World One Meal At A Time

# J.F. PARKER

# BOOK DESCRIPTION

Imagine the impact changing your diet could have on your well-being and the world as we know it. Have you ever felt a strong desire to contribute to the environment in a positive way, but didn't know where to begin? Adopting an environmentally conscious diet may be the answer, as it could help achieve both of these goals simultaneously.

By following a plant-based, vegan, or vegetarian diet, you can greatly benefit mind, body, and spirit, while also creating a better world for the future of humanity and our Earth.

Did you know that the United States could decrease greenhouse gas emissions by 82 million metric tons per year by reducing the consumption of meat by only 25% and substituting this with plant proteins? This is just one statistic resulting from a single study...

**Getting started may seem difficult, but by knowing more and doing more, the impact you could make on the environment and your health has no bounds.**

The following material is meant to guide you in your journey towards an environmentally friendly and health-conscious lifestyle for the foreseeable future. Inside *Plant-Based, Vegetarian, and Vegan Diets for Beginners*, you will learn:

- About the background and benefits of plant-based, vegetarian, and vegan diets

- About the studies, research and real-life accounts on the effects of plant-based, vegetarian and vegan diets
- About the effects, a plant-based, vegetarian or vegan diet has on the environment.

**How to live a healthier and richer life by following a plant-based, vegetarian, or vegan diet**

You will learn and discover so much more!

This book will expand your knowledge and give you the tools to live a healthier lifestyle. Who knew you could help the world and others by making a few changes to your diet?

**Make a change by fueling your mind and body, and protecting the earth with the power of *Plant-Based, Vegetarian, and Vegan Diets for Beginners*!**

# TABLE OF CONTENTS

# INTRODUCTION

This book will guide you towards the transformation of your mind and body through the exploration and investigation of plant-based, vegetarian, and vegan diets. Utilizing a holistic approach, we will address multiple aspects of each diet. The following information is intended to inform, educate and inspire openness in consideration of practicing an alternative lifestyle. We will discuss the definitions, backgrounds, and implications of each diet while considering the academic research and scientific studies behind them.

The following information will work to provide different views of plant-based, vegetarian, and vegan diets in a realistic and idealistic manner. We will discuss the benefits and risks involved when employing each of these three diets — not only will we look at the effects on personal health of these diets, but also the potential environmental outcomes of them. This book will provide possible avenues and approaches to take to help you decide for yourself whether a change in your diet is desirable. This book is a guide, but the journey is still yours.

We will consider the facts and opinions on plant-based, vegetarian, and vegan diets, as well as answer some commonly held questions. The freedom to contemplate, explore, and investigate various paths to an alternative lifestyle is imperative. It is possible to make a positive change, live a more ethical life, and help benefit the planet by being more conscious of your consumption. The information provided is intended to help you decide which lifestyle is in alignment with your goals. These three diets are not one-size-fits-all diets; you need to listen to your own mind and body when determining if one of these lifestyles is right for you.

It is apparent that learning to look after our bodies, minds, and homes may be put on the back-burner frequently given the happenings of everyday life. The busyness of trying to keep up with work, family, and relationships often restricts us from prioritizing and taking care of ourselves. The desire to lead a fuller and healthier life may be the reason we push ourselves out of our comfort zones. Others may be seeking inspiration or knowledge alone... Let us go on this journey together with mindfulness, openness, and kindness for all bodies and living creatures. This guide will ultimately help you to expand your knowledge and inspire hope for not only the future, but for that of the great provisions and capabilities of our Earth.

## Overview

This guide has been divided into three parts: the plant-based diet, the vegetarian diet, and the vegan diet. All will be equitably discussed and examined to provide accurate and compelling information. Comparing and contrasting the different diets and lifestyles will grant a deeper understanding of the effects these diets have on our bodies and our planet. We will explore the diets based on what we have learned from studies and experiences thus far and we will also look at how you can tailor these diets to your specific needs and lifestyle.

Chapters 1 through 3 are purely dedicated to the plant-based diet. In these chapters, we discuss the background and concept of the plant-based diet, as well as examples and the effects this diet has or could have on your health and the environment. This will be supported by case studies, research, and shared personal accounts — some frequently asked questions will be also answered in order to clear up some common confusion or debates around plant-based diets.

In chapters 4 through 6, we will delve into the vegetarian diet. These chapters will discuss and define the vegetarian diet with the help of many academic studies. This will form the foundation for the rest of our discussion on the health and environmental effects of the vegetarian diet. Examples of vegetarian meals will be provided as well. Real accounts and case studies that reveal how the vegetarian diet can be modified and unique to each person will be assessed,. This works to remind us that every person's body and experience is different. Lastly, some popular questions about the vegetarian diet will also be answered.

Finally, the third section of this book will discuss the fast-growing and trending vegan diet. Chapters 7, 8, and 9 go into further detail about this more restrictive diet and all-encompassing lifestyle. We will look at some examples of vegan meals and some specific vegan lifestyle criteria. We will then discuss the potential health and environmental effects of this lifestyle before answering some of the frequently asked questions surrounding the diet. In conclusion, there will be discussion of the contents within the previous 9 chapters, focussing on the meanings, differences, effects, and implications of all three diets.

# CHAPTER 1

# THE PLANT-BASED DIET EXPLAINED

## What Is a Plant-Based Diet?

### Defining a Plant-Based Diet

There has been a rise in the use of the word "plant-based" in recent years; we see it used as a marketing tactic on product labels, on social media and cooking channels, and even in descriptions on modern restaurant menus. Although this word has become quite popular among people today, the general public tends to not know exactly what this means. There is a need to define the "plant-based" diet to prevent misuse, misinterpretation, and the spread of misinformation about this particular lifestyle.

The plant-based diet consists of "raw" or minimally processed fruit, vegetables, legumes, and grains, while excluding or minimizing animal products such as meats, poultry, eggs, seafood, and dairy products. This diet is also associated with "raw" or "whole" foods. This means that the foods and ingredients one eats when following this diet have fewer additives and preservatives, and are often organic or true to their natural grown form. The idea of "plant" in a plant-based diet is key to understanding this specific diet. An individual following this diet relies on plants and whole foods to meet their daily and nutritional requirements, rather than packed and processed foods that consist of animal products and manufactured ingredients.

The plant-based diet is naturally centralized on plants, and involves incorporating more foods grown from the Earth while excluding or minimizing processed foods like animal products that are refined, high in fat, and cholesterol-dense. This involves the consumption of mostly organic and naturally produced plants — anything edible and nutritious grown from the soil — with occasional or almost no animal products, like yogurt or kefir, fish, eggs and poultry, and lean meats. Those who follow a plant-based diet often view it as returning to our original roots as homo-sapiens.

### *Plant-Based Meal Ideas*

Now that we know what following a plant-based diet entails, let us look at some examples of plant-based meals. These menus will include meals solely made out of plants and grains, as well as meals that are plant-focused with additional animal products providing healthy fats and high protein. Before we dive right in, we need to be aware of the nutritional value of plant-based meals, so that we do not follow a plant-based diet blindly.

The three macronutrients human bodies need are carbohydrates, proteins, and fats. Our bodies rely heavily on these three main nutrients, and when we do not consume enough of any one of them, our bodies will suffer and become deficient in many micronutrients as well. It is recommended by many doctors and dietitians that the average person's total daily calories need to be made up of 45%-65% carbohydrates,

20%-30% fats, and 10%-30% protein (Ryan-Harshman and Aldoori, 2006). The amount of energy our bodies 'need varies based on weight, age, height, genetics, and physical activity. Therefore, you would need to tailor these meals to your body's unique needs, which can be done by observing your energy and mood levels throughout the day, alongside your hunger cues and following your doctor's or dietitian's advice.

According to multiple thorough scientific and medical studies, the recommended caloric intake for an adult male is 2,500 calories per day, while an adult female's is 2000 calories. This is an average estimate based on studies, observations, and personal experiences that have been shared throughout recent history.

Here are some plant-based meals that exclude animal products:

| Meal | Ingredients |
| --- | --- |
| **Breakfast** | Oat Bowl:<br>½ dry oats<br>¼ oat milk<br>1 tbsp nut butter (your preference)<br>1 banana<br>1 tbsp hemp seeds<br>1 tbsp maple syrup<br>Nutrition:<br>533kcal<br>81.4g total carbohydrates<br>19.5g protein<br>22.8g total fats |

| | |
|---|---|
| **Lunch** | Chickpea-<br><br>Avocado Smash:<br><br>½ cup canned chickpeas<br><br>½ avocado<br><br>2 slices toast (your preference)<br><br>1 tbsp nutritional yeast flakes<br><br>Nutrition:<br><br>532kcal<br><br>64.5g total carbohydrates<br><br>18.8g protein<br><br>25.6g total fats |
| **Dinner** | Lentil Stew:<br><br>1 cup cooked lentils<br><br>1 cup cooked mixed vegetables (your preference)<br><br>½ cooked spinach<br><br>1 cup cooked quinoa<br><br>1 tbsp nutritional yeast flakes<br><br>Nutrition:<br><br>525kcal<br><br>136.3g total carbohydrates<br><br>42.6g protein<br><br>17.2g total fats |

Here are examples of plant-based meals that include animal products:

| Meal | Ingredients |
|---|---|
| **Breakfast** | Yogurt Bowl:<br><br>1 cup of Greek yogurt<br><br>½ cup fresh mixed berries<br><br>¼ mixed nuts<br><br>1 tbsp raw honey<br><br>Nutrition:<br><br>513kcal<br><br>33.5g total carbohydrates<br><br>26.5g protein<br><br>26.3g total fats |
| **Lunch** | Egg and Avocado Toast:<br><br>2 Slices of bread (your preference)<br><br>2 eggs<br><br>½ an avocado<br><br>Nutrition:<br><br>505kcal<br><br>40.1g total carbohydrates<br><br>22.9g protein<br><br>32.1g total fats |

| **Dinner** | Salmon and Salad: |
|---|---|
| | 1 sustainably sourced salmon steak (4 ounces) |
| | 1 cup of baby spinach |
| | ½ cup of cherry tomatoes |
| | ½ cup cubed cucumber |
| | ½ spiralized carrots |
| | ¼ avocado |
| | 1 tbsp balsamic vinegar |
| | Nutrition: |
| | 329kcal |
| | 19.7g total carbohydrates |
| | 33g protein |
| | 14.6g total fats |

The nutritional values have been calculated using the mobile application Lose It!™

## What We Know About Plant-Based Diets

### *Studies on the Plant-Based Diet*

Although we have seen an increase in the talk and research on plant-based diets, this diet has not been fully adopted worldwide. An interesting 2015 study done by Pohjolainen, Vinnari and Jokinen displayed consumer's reasons behind the challenges of following a plant-based diet. The scholars 'work, published by the British Food Journal, revealed that the major barriers to following a plant-based diet were the enjoyment of meat, people's eating routines, health ideologies, and the difficulties involved with the preparation of vegetarian food.

Furthermore, the scholars observed the socio-demographics, values, and meat consumption frequency of their study's population. They discovered that the barriers to following a plant-based diet correlated with factors that fell under either socio-demographics, values, or meat consumption frequency. These factors included being a man, being of a younger age, living in a rural residence, living in a household with children, having low or poor education, having no exposure to vegetarianism through a vegetarian friend or family member, or valuing traditions and wealth associated with high meat consumption.

The study's findings showed that education, cultural norms and traditions, and accessibility were the main issues and social barriers to following a plant-based diet. The scholars provided suggestions to increase the adoption of plant-based diets, given the dangerous health and environmental implications of high meat consumption. One of these suggestions was changing the meals provided at public school cafeterias and canteens, which would then increase the accessibility of plant-based diets among the youth — the scholars then suggested that schools shift to more plant-based meals by increasing vegetarian foods in school meals, therefore decreasing one perceived barrier to following a plant-based diet. The scholars' work is one small but significant example of how a person and a community can transform their eating behavior to benefit their health and their environment.

## FAQ: The Plant-Based Diet Explained

### How can a plant-based diet be sustainable for me?

You can be well-prepared before you start the diet; try to educate yourself on plant-based foods, as well as your personal health and nutritional needs. You should also know whether you can adjust your time, energy, and finances to follow a plant-based diet. You need to ask yourself whether you have access to plenty of plant-based foods, and if your nutritional needs can be met if you follow this diet.

### Will a plant-based diet prolong my life?

A plant-based diet could potentially improve your health, further preventing you from acquiring any diseases that could shorten your life. In this guide, we look at many studies that show how a plant-based diet can prevent one from suffering from hypertension, high blood pressure, high cholesterol, type 2 diabetes, obesity, and some cancers.

### Can my children follow a plant-based diet as well?

Yes, as it is best to act as a model for your children. Children copy our habits and daily behaviors, and even our eating habits — if your children are receiving enough calories, macronutrients, and micronutrients for their growth and development, they can definitely follow a plant-based diet with you. Remember to allow your children to try new foods, and to also give them the freedom to adjust their diet according to their needs.

### Is a plant-based diet a diet of only plants?

No. A plant-based diet can include the occasional consumption of sustainable and ethically sourced animal products, like meats, seafood, or poultry. A plant-based diet can also exclude animal products, consisting of only fruits, vegetables, grains, and legumes.

## Chapter Summary: The Plant-Based Diet Explained

In this first chapter, we explained and defined the plant-based diet, made of whole organic foods with minimal processed animal products. Meal plans which you can try out were also provided as inspiration, and we can now see just how easy and affordable it is to incorporate more fresh fruits and vegetables into our diets. We also looked at the plant-based diet from an academic perspective by discussing a study done by Pohjolainen, Vinnari and Jokinen on the accessibility and potential benefits of the plant-based diet among a particular community. We also answered some frequently asked questions that often circulate around recent discussions on the plant-based diet.

Some lessons we learned from this chapter:

- The plant-based diet is a diet that consists of organic and whole foods, with little to no animal products and processed foods.
- A great plant-based food source you can incorporate into your diet is oats, as it consists of an affordable and accessible grain packed with great nutrients like fiber for fullness and satiation.
- We can promote a more plant-based lifestyle through inspiring and educating our community and youth of today.

# CHAPTER 2

# THE PLANT-BASED DIET AND YOUR HEALTH

## The Effects of Plant-Based Diets on Your Health Explained

The plant-based diet has become popular in recent years, especially in the health and fitness community. Due to the convenience, affordability, and accessibility of fast foods — which are high in calories, saturated fats, sodium, and preservatives — we have seen an increase in obesity, as well as other health problems and concerns like heart disease and type 2 diabetes. Many healthcare professionals have advised their patients to incorporate more plants into their diets, cutting out meats and animal products. The lack of fresh whole foods has been one of main causes of our health issues today, along with stress levels.

Therefore, the plant-based diet can act as a remedy to this global health issue. By following a more plant-oriented diet, you are filling and fueling your body with the nutrients it needs to function optimally. Plant-based diets are usually focused on whole and raw produce, which is less processed and has no additives. Many people who are health-conscious enjoy this diet because they know what is in their food, and therefore have peace of mind by knowing what nutrients they are getting or not getting. The physical, emotional, and psychological effects of a plant-based diet are clear, as is the link between these effects; if one knows they are eating nutritious and better quality food, they will feel better about their actions, and their ego will receive a boost while their body receives a boost of nutrient-dense and healthy food. This further improves its performance, which will then improve the person's view of themself.

Observing how to live on plant-based foods will change your perspective on food and nutrition, as you will become more aware of what you put in your body and how you treat it. The change in mood and physical effects are evident — to demonstrate this, eat a fast food meal for lunch and monitor the way your mind and body feels, even going as far as writing down your experience. For your next meal, eat a balanced plant-based diet that includes fresh vegetables, some grains, and a sustainable high-quality protein source. Observe the way you feel after the meal, as well as for the rest of the evening. You should be able to compare the two meal experiences and identify the difference in energy and mood, as well as digestion and satiation.

When following a plant-based diet, one needs to be aware of some nutrients you might be missing out on, especially if you are excluding meats. People that do not get enough iron can be at risk of being deficient in iron, which often results in the decrease of red blood cells needed to carry oxygen around our body. This disorder is known as anemia. A person who has low iron and therefore low red blood cell levels, often feel tired, weak and appear pale, but the health risks of low iron can result in more serious complications if not treated as our bodies need oxygen to function. Another health issue concerning red blood cells is the condition known as Macrocytosis or megaloblastic anemia, where red blood cells are larger than normal (Vega, Younes, and Kuriakose, 2008). This condition is associated with genetics and lifestyle, specifically the deficiency of vitamin B-12 which can occur when following a plant-based diet that excludes animal products and B-12 supplements.

The many effects of following a plant-based diet have been monitored by dietitians and researchers, and findings have shown how a plant-based diet can prevent or aid in fighting against many health conditions and diseases. Kathleen E. Allen, Divya Gumber, and Robert J. Ostfeld have studied the positive effects that following a plant-based diet can have on a person's health, especially someone who has health conditions like heart disease, diabetes or obesity (Allen, Gumber, and Ostfeld, 2019). Health issues like inflammation, hypertension, indigestion, high levels of cholesterol and saturated fats, and diseases like obesity and diabetes were studied by these three researchers, and they identified there was a correlation between each issue and a plant-based diet.

The researchers explain that diets high in animal products increase serum levels of inflammation, whereas a diet with fewer animal products like a plant-based diet will lower the serum levels of inflammation. Hypertension, on the other hand, is caused by high blood pressure, so following a plant-based diet lowers blood pressure — this is due to higher potassium intake, decreased sodium intake, and improvement in blood vessel dilation, among other chemical processes. The plant-based diet has been associated with lower systolic and diastolic blood pressure, which aids in the prevention of hypertension. Another potential positive effect of following a plant-based diet is the improvement in digestion, which is due to the changes of the microbiome in the digestive system. Due to the increase in soluble dietary fiber seen in the plant-based diet, the bacteria in the colon is nourished, which allows it to produce short-chain fatty acids instead of long-chain fatty acids. The difference in these chains is ultimately the reason why people who follow a plant-based diet can have lower cholesterol, as this can prevent coronary artery disease and myocardial infarction, or heart attack.

Furthermore, because of the reduction in animal fat and overproduced foods, the plant-based diet results in lower serum lipid levels due to low saturated fat and high soluble fiber intake. Certain healthy plant-based fats, like almond or pistachio nuts, may reduce levels of high-density lipoprotein, which has been associated with high cholesterol. We can see that the replacement of animal fats with healthy nuts and seed-sourced fats in a plant-based diet results in significant health effects, both present and future. These also further reduce a person from overeating or consuming too many unhealthy fats that cause obesity. Another disease that can be treated or prevented by the plant-based diet is diabetes, which is caused by the lack of insulin in the body. Most of the time, both type 1 and 2 diabetes are strongly connected to diet. Whether it is due to high levels of added-sugar and excessive carbohydrates that worsen symptoms of diabetes due to high blood sugar levels, or simply genetic, one needs to learn how to manage the disease. One way is to transform your diet into a low-sugar and low-carbohydrate diet. Your body struggles to convert sugar into energy without insulin, but research suggests that following a plant-based diet can actually aid in insulin sensitivity (Allen, Gumber, and Ostfeld, 2019).

Despite the more serious health issues that plant-based diets can aid or alleviate, the diet is still beneficial for people without these diseases. The plant-based diet has been used as one form of treatment for heart disease, obesity, and diabetes, but can also be followed without urgency or necessity. Unlike vegetarian diets, this diet is more focused on the quality of food and the balance of the food on your plate — it is also less restrictive, as it can include high-quality meat like salmon or free-range chicken. For people who would like to transform the way they think, feel, and act, a plant-based diet is a step in the right direction to reap many health benefits from natural food.

***The Health Benefits of Following a Plant-Based Diet***

- Lower risk of heart disease
- Low body mass index (BMI)
- Low cholesterol levels
- Low risk of obesity
- Low risk of diabetes
- Lower blood pressure
- Lower risk of colon cancer
- Improvement in digestion

***The Health Risks of Following a Plant-Based Diet***

- Low BMI
- B12 Deficiency
- Zinc Deficiency
- Iron Deficiency (Heme Iron)
- Potential Anemia
- Potential Macrocytosis

## A Case Study: The Plant-Based Diet and Your Health

A study on the health and transformation of a middle-aged obese woman was reviewed by Allen, Gumber, and Ostfeld in 2019. The study focused on the correlation between following a plant-based diet and the changes and health improvements of the 54-year-old woman, who suffered from grade 4 obesity as well as type 2 diabetes. At the beginning of the study, the woman was in an unhealthy state, with a body mass index (BMI) OF 45.2 kg/m².

The study followed and observed the woman's progress. The woman started out as overweight with type 2 diabetes, as well as lower extremity edema on her left side. After seeing a physician and taking tests, it was discovered that the woman had experienced heart failure, as well as a depressed left ventricular systolic function. Both the woman's heart and her life were in danger; from this diagnosis, it became clear that she needed to change her lifestyle, especially when it came to her diet. Her diet was a "western diet", which is very accepted in most Western societies. This diet could seem balanced, but there are many unknown additives and additional nutrients like sodium, fat, and calories. These are all essential to the human body's diet, but when we consume high amounts of these regularly, it can be detrimental to our health. An excess of anything good can be bad, so the key to good health is *balance*. A natural and balanced whole food plant-based diet is what the woman had to start following in order to improve her health, ultimately saving her life.

The woman followed a plant-based diet while also taking vitamin B-12 supplements. She had lost 48.5 pounds in this period, and she was also able to reverse her diabetes without using diabetes medications. In addition to following a plant-based diet, the woman also received medical heart therapy for her heart failure. After consistently implementing these two forms of treatment for just under 6 months, the woman had experienced great results and improvement in her health. Another positive result from this diet and lifestyle change was that her left ventricular systolic function had normalized (Allen, Gumber, and Ostfeld, 2019).

This case study of one single woman's health journey, which resulted in positive health changes, gives us a glimpse of the possible health benefits that many more people could receive from following a plant-based diet. Again, you do not need to be ill or unhealthy to start following a plant-based diet — you can start and follow a plant-based diet whenever you want and however you want, as long as you are getting all your nutritional needs met. Your diet cannot fix all your life problems, but it can definitely give your life a physical, emotional, and psychological boost.

## FAQ: The Plant-Based Diet and Your Health

### Can I still gain muscle on a plant-based diet?

You can gain muscle on a plant-based diet by incorporating more protein in your diet, or add plant protein powders to your smoothies or meals to boost your protein intake. Remember, in addition to following a protein-rich plant-based diet, you need to exercise regularly with muscle-building techniques.

### Will my old age make it challenging for me to follow a plant-based diet?

You can adjust or change your diet in small or big ways. If your health has been affected by your age, especially old age, you should consult your general practitioner or dietician before transitioning to a plant-based diet. You should be aware of your unique nutritional needs before starting a new plant-based diet, despite the many health benefits and various nutrients it can provide.

**Do I still need to be taking multivitamins on a plant-based diet?**

If you feel any new symptoms like fatigue, or if your energy and concentration levels are dropping, you should speak to your doctor. You can be tested for nutrient deficiencies, which will help you be aware of any supplements you might need to take; a vital supplement for a plant-based diet that excludes meat is a vitamin B-12 supplement.

**How do I know if I am getting enough nutrients and macronutrients from my plant-based diet?**

You can make an appointment with your doctor to test for any deficiencies. You can also download a nutrition app to log your daily meals and track your calorie, protein, fat, and carbohydrate intake.

## Chapter Summary: The Plant-Based Diet and Your Health

In this chapter, we focused on the many health-related factors involved with the implementation of a plant-based diet. In this discussion, we looked at the potential health benefits and health risks a plant-based diet could pose on a person's body, encouraging contemplation and interest in the ways it could influence your well-being. We then considered a case study done by Allen, Gumber, and Ostfeld that discussed the health effects of a plant-based diet on an unhealthy middle-aged woman. This case study proved to only highlight the health benefits of the plant-based diet — while this was an extreme case, we could see how changing your diet truly does change your overall well-being. Some lessons we learned from this chapter:

- The plant-based diet can prevent many health issues like diabetes, high and dangerous cholesterol levels, and obesity.

- The plant-based diet should be accompanied by other lifestyle changes to reap the best results for your health.

- You can and should adjust your plant-based diet to your personal health and nutritional needs.

# CHAPTER 3

# THE PLANT-BASED DIET AND THE ENVIRONMENT

## The Effects of a Plant-Based Diet on the Environment Explained

More and more people have started to follow a plant-based diet in recent years, due to both the health changes and benefits of the diet and the reduction of the consumption of animal products. The latter has to do with the environmental effects of the typical "western diet", which has been promoted, exported and advertised across the globe. Due to easier and more accessible travel as well as the internet, people from different countries have been exchanging ideas and attitudes, and this includes ideas and attitudes around food.

The 20th century saw the boom of fast food and factory-made processed products. Convenience foods were on the rise as people's lifestyles shifted; the influence of American culture and the "American dream" only grew and stretched wider than ever before via television, Hollywood, and frequent traveling. The idea of fast-food and a big portion of affordable and tasty meals was accepted with open arms, as most of these fast-food chains serve affordable meals that contain animal products and preservatives to enhance flavor, enjoyment, and shelf life of their foods. While this global food phenomenon was widely accepted by many countries, the effects of packaged, fast food, and processed foods were only experienced and discovered later. We only see the long-term effects of our everyday habits after the fact, sometimes when it is too late.

With the culture of convenience and fast-paced lifestyles came the demand for fast and convenient food. We want what we cannot have, and we also want what we want as soon as possible; the impatience and selfishness of human nature has been catered for and encouraged by the mass production of food. In the last few decades, we have seen how humankind has turned a necessity — food — into a luxury and a desire. There have been major consequences of this global food production machine, as both the health of the population and the planet have been compromised. The environmental effects of mass production and consumption of manufactured food have been increasing, and have now taken a turn for the worst.

Now that we have lived through the boom of mass food production and its negative effects on our planet, many of us have become educated in how and where we can eat our food. We want to know the carbon footprint of the steak on our plate, or of the brightly packaged candy bar we had for an afternoon snack. These contemplations have led to more people transforming the way they consume and eat, cutting down on packaged and processed convenience foods both for their health and for the environment.

Therefore, following a plant-based diet can be one step in the direction of changing the way we produce and consume. If there is no demand, there will be no supply — if we begin to buy more fresh vegetables than beef jerky sticks, we will change the course of food production. The production of meat requires more resources than the production of plants, grains and legumes, meaning that we will waste less energy and produce less carbon dioxide into the atmosphere. When we plant fruit-bearing trees, we will provide more oxygen for humans and the creatures around us, but if we farm more cows, we will provide more methane, threatening the air we and other animals breathe while also contributing to the damage done to the ozone layer. If we reduce our consumption and production of meat and animal products, we will reduce the resources needed for that production. A 2019 study done by Eshel, Stainier, Shepon, and Swaminathan presents the potential benefits of plant-based production by comparing the current state of animal produce farms; the study highlights the benefits of farming plant-based products, as well as the environmental effects of replacing meat with plant alternatives like legumes and tofu. The authors 'work states that if American change their diets, replacing meat with plant alternatives, less pastureland will be used and more cropland can be grown. This ultimately means that there will be less methane and greenhouse gas emissions, while irrigation needs for cropland will increase by 15% (Eshel et al., 2019).

Although shifting one's diet and society's consumption is challenging at first, plant-based products can ultimately reduce our carbon footprint, as they will reduce the known causes of global warming and climate change: mass farming, production and exportation of animal products.

## The Positive Environmental Effects of a Plant-Based Diet

- Reduction of greenhouse gases

- Less need and usage of fossil fuels

- A reduction in the risk of animal-borne diseases

- An increase in organic and ethically grown products

- A reduction in genetically modified organisms (GMOs), mono-cultivation (farming one crop or product at a time), and preservatives

- A reduction of plastic use

- A reduction of air, water, and land pollution

*The Negative Environmental Effects of a Plant-Based Diet*

- Potential harm on plant diversity and plant life

- The increase in alien invasive plants

- Soil and land erosion

## A Case Study: The Plant-Based Diet and the Environment

A 2018 study done by van de Kamp and Temme observes the ways people choose their meals, looking at the effects on nutrition, the environment, and the taste of different lunch meals at a specific workplace. The study looked at the buffet-style lunch that was served at a workplace, which consisted of three types of meals: animal-based foods, plant-based foods, and combinations of both. All employees at the workplace had a choice between these three types of meals.

The employees then had to score the three different meals from 1 to 10, based on the food's taste and their appreciation for the food. Meanwhile, the researchers were studying other elements of the food, such as the environmental impact each meal had, the nutritional intake of each meal, and the appreciation and tastiness of each meal. These were determined by the ingredients of the meals, as well as the opinions of the employees. The researchers also used life cycle assessments to calculate the greenhouse gas emissions that each buffet contributed.

The results and findings of the study showed that the plant-based and combination meal scored higher in tastiness than the animal-based meal. The plant-based diet lunch had the lowest score in terms of greenhouse gas emissions and land use, while the animal-based lunch had the highest. With regards to nutritional intake, the animal-based lunch had the highest level of saturated fat, while the combination lunch was seen to have more fiber but less saturated fat and more energy intake. Interestingly, the plant-based diet did not increase energy intake, but did increase fiber intake while decreasing both sodium and saturated fat intakes. From these results, van de Kamp and Temme concluded that plant-based diets can be tasty and nutritious for the general public, while stabilizing energy and calorie levels and possessing the lowest impact on the environment out of all the diets (van de Kamp and Temme, 2018).

# FAQ: The Plant-based Diet and the Environment

**Are free-range chicken eggs better than battery farmed chicken eggs?**

Yes. Battery chickens are kept in harsh conditions and are mistreated. Free-range chickens are left to roam and graze outside and not forced into a tiny cage or given hormones.

**Is organic food better for the environment?**

Yes. Organically grown produce does not involve dangerous pesticides or other manufactured chemicals that harm the natural ecosystems and plant life around the cropland.

**How do I know if the fish that I am eating has been ethically and sustainably sourced?**

You can look at the packaging of the fish for a logo or sticker that certifies the product as "sustainably sourced". You can also go to your local fish markets or fishermen and buy fresh fish — this way, your carbon footprint is reduced, as no plastic packaging or transportation is involved.

**Is a plant-based diet better for the environment than a vegetarian diet?**

A plant-based diet involves fewer processes and packaged ingredients, while a vegetarian diet still consists of processed plant-based and animal-based products. Both the plant-based diet and the vegetarian diet can benefit the environment; you can purchase locally sourced and free-range animal products, or keep reusable containers or shopping bags. Your diet is just one of many ways you can help protect the planet.

## Chapter Summary: The Plant-Based Diet and the Environment

This chapter explored the relationship between the plant-based diet and the environment. The very prevalent environmental issues of today were discussed, along with ways we can go about preventing these issues from continuing to harm our planet. The plant-based diet was viewed as a way to counteract the atrocities caused by the mass production of many packaged, processed, and animal products. The culture and attitudes of people were highlighted and deemed as one of the contributing factors to the food industries' environmentally harmful and unethical practices. An example of how this counteraction occurs was shown in the case study by van de Kamp and Temme, who saw how people enjoy choice, variety, and convenience during work lunchtime. This only worked to show how humans enjoy choice and the sense of agency, even when it comes to lunch at work.

Some lessons we learned in this chapter:

- With more people following a plant-based diet, we could reduce the amount of greenhouse gas emissions.

- Marketing and presentation are important drivers in people choosing a plant-based diet over another diet.

- Cultural norms, values, and attitudes concerning food need to change for the plant-based diet to become more popular, and therefore a significant and real solution to climate change.

# CHAPTER 4

# THE VEGETARIAN DIET EXPLAINED

## What is a Vegetarian Diet?

### Defining a Vegetarian Diet

The vegetarian diet can be defined as a diet that excludes any meat, poultry, or seafood. Although there are many different ways people follow a vegetarian diet, there are five different types of vegetarian diets primarily followed by people today. These five types of diets are:

1. Total vegetarian, or vegan: A diet that excludes meat, poultry, and seafood, as well as animal products and by-products like eggs, dairy products, gelatin, and even honey.
2. Lacto-ovo vegetarian: A diet that excludes meat, poultry, and seafood, but includes eggs and dairy products
3. Lacto-vegetarian: A diet that excludes meat, poultry, seafood, and eggs, but includes dairy products
4. Ovo-vegetarian: A diet that excludes meat, poultry, and seafood, but includes eggs

5.  Partial vegetarian, or flexitarian: A diet that excludes meat, but might include poultry (pollo-vegetarian) or seafood (pesco-vegetarian or pescatarian)

Although there has been a growing number of vegetarians across the globe — especially in Western societies — most people still incorporate meat into their diet. In countries like India, the religious practice of certain Hindi sects is the reason behind more people excluding meat from their diet. Aside from these religious influences, the recent increase of vegetarianism in the West is also associated with access to education, as well as the freedom and privilege of choice. Many areas and countries across the globe do not have the means to follow restricted diets, as the main goal is to consume enough calories to survive. When following a diet of restriction, one needs to have the means, time, and information accessible to them in order to follow the diet that restricts without losing out on any vital nutrients. This skill can be quite challenging, even for people who have the means and opportunities to follow a vegetarian diet. Due to the fact that there are different types of vegetarian diets, we need to be conscious of how these diets are different in foods as well as nutrients; some vegetarian diets are less restrictive than others, while some are easier and less expensive to maintain.

This reality means that one can and should follow a vegetarian diet according to their nutritional needs, cultural, and personal preferences, as well as their financial situation. One's body and one's budget need to be addressed when planning a vegetarian menu; while plants are often cheaper and tax-free in most countries, the nutrients and satiation they provide will not be the same as meat products. As such, we need to educate ourselves on the general nutrition, price and accessibility of the foods we consume.

## *Vegetarian Meal Ideas*

Here are some examples of vegetarian meals, beginning with total vegetarian:

| Meal | Ingredients |
|---|---|
| **Breakfast** | Protein Oat Bowl:<br><br>½ cup dry oats<br><br>1 heaped scoop protein powder<br><br>1 banana<br><br>1 tbsp nut butter (your preference)<br><br>1 tbsp hemp seeds<br><br>1 tbsp maple syrup<br><br>Nutrition:<br><br>645kcal<br><br>131.8g total carbohydrates<br><br>38.3g protein<br><br>23g total fats |

| Lunch | Vegan Toasted Cheese with Side Salad:<br>2 slices bread (your preference)<br>2 slices of vegan cheddar cheese<br>1/2 cup butter lettuce<br>½ cherry tomatoes<br>½ sliced cucumber<br>¼ raw coleslaw<br>⅛ cup red onion<br>¼ cooked beetroot<br>1 tbsp balsamic vinegar<br>Nutrition:<br>327kcal<br>36.5g total carbohydrates<br>10.4g protein<br>13.7g total fats |
|---|---|
| **Dinner** | Tofu Stir Fry:<br>1 cup cubed firm tofu<br>1 cup raw coleslaw<br>½ sliced bell peppers<br>1 cherry tomatoes<br>¼ sliced onion<br>1 cup spinach<br>1 tbsp low sodium soy sauce<br>Nutrition:<br>234kcal<br>30.4g total carbohydrates<br>20.1g protein<br>10.7g total fats |

Lacto-ovo vegetarian meals :

| Meal | Ingredients |
| --- | --- |
| **Breakfast** | Eggs on Toast:<br>2 slices bread (your preference)<br>2 eggs<br>¼ cup sliced tomato<br>¼ arugula<br>Nutrition:<br>279kcal<br>29.7g total carbohydrates<br>12.6g protein<br>11.4g total fats |
| **Lunch** | Mediterranean Salad:<br>1 cup canned chickpeas<br>½ cup cubed cucumber<br>½ cubed tomato<br>¼ crumbled feta cheese<br>1 tbsp extra virgin olive oil<br>1 tbsp balsamic vinegar<br>1 tsp lemon juice<br>Nutrition:<br>539kcal<br>62.2g total carbohydrates<br>18.4g protein<br>25.2g total fats |

| Dinner | Pesto Pasta: <br> 1 cup of cooked pasta (your preference) <br> ½ cherry tomatoes <br> ¼ cubed mozzarella cheese <br> 1 tbsp basil pesto <br> Nutrition: <br> 377kcal <br> 48.8g total carbohydrates <br> 15.7g protein <br> 12.8 total fats |
|---|---|

Lacto-vegetarian meals :

| Meal | Ingredients |
|---|---|
| Breakfast | Yogurt Bowl: <br> 1 cup plain yogurt <br> ½ mixed fruit <br> ¼ mixed nuts <br> 1 tbsp maple syrup <br> 1 tsp cinnamon <br> Nutrition: <br> 480kcal <br> 39.5g total carbohydrates <br> 18.5g protein <br> 28.1g total fats |

| | |
|---|---|
| **Lunch** | Toasted Cheese with Side Salad:<br><br>2 slices bread (your preference)<br><br>2 slices cheddar cheese<br><br>1 cup baby spinach<br><br>½ cherry tomatoes<br><br>½ sliced cucumber<br><br>¼ grated carrot<br><br>1 tbsp of dressing (your preference)<br><br>Nutrition:<br><br>406kcal<br><br>31.8g total carbohydrates<br><br>23.4g protein<br><br>24.6g total fats |
| **Dinner** | Lentil Cottage Pie:<br><br>1 cup cooked lentils<br><br>½ cooked mixed vegetables<br><br>1 cup mashed potatoes<br><br>¼ grated cheddar cheese<br><br>Nutrition:<br><br>517kcal<br><br>82.7g total carbohydrates<br><br>31.5g protein<br><br>19.8g total fats |

Ovo-vegetarian meals:

| Meal | Ingredients |
| --- | --- |
| **Breakfast** | Oat Flapjacks:<br>1 cup dry oats<br>1 ½ cup almond milk<br>1 egg<br>1 tsp baking soda<br>1 tsp vanilla extract<br>½ mixed berries<br>1 tbsp maple syrup<br>Nutrition:<br>572kcal<br>87.4g total carbohydrates<br>20g protein<br>13.8g total fats |
| **Lunch** | Poached Eggs on Avocado Toast:<br>2 slices bread (your preference)<br>2 eggs<br>½ avocado<br>1 tbsp nutritional yeast flakes<br>Nutrition:<br>520kcal<br>41.4g total carbohydrates<br>24.9g protein<br>32.2g total fats |

| Dinner | Chickpea Curry: |
|---|---|
| | 1 cup canned chickpeas |
| | 1 cup cooked mixed vegetables |
| | 1 tsp curry powder |
| | 1 cup cooked brown rice |
| | Nutrition: |
| | 651kcal |
| | 112.7g total carbohydrates |
| | 20g protein |
| | 13.3g total fats |

Partial vegetarian meals:

| Meal | Ingredients |
|---|---|
| Breakfast | Breakfast Wrap: |
| | 1 wheat tortilla wrap |
| | 2 eggs |
| | 1 slice cheddar cheese |
| | ¼ sliced tomato |
| | ⅛ cup sliced onion |
| | Nutrition: |
| | 358kcal |
| | 29.9g total carbohydrates |
| | 21.6g protein |
| | 17,8g total fats |

| | |
|---|---|
| **Lunch** | Vegetable Tacos:<br>2 corn taco shells<br>½ sliced cos lettuce<br>½ cubed tomatoes<br>¼ grated cheddar cheese<br>½ soy mince<br>4 tbsp guacamole<br>4 tbsp salsa dressing<br>Nutrition:<br>453kcal<br>36,8g total carbohydrates<br>24.3g protein<br>65g total fats |
| **Dinner** | Smoked Chicken Salad:<br>1 cup shredded smoked chicken<br>1 cup baby spinach<br>½ cherry tomatoes<br>½ sliced cucumber<br>¼ grated carrot<br>⅛ red onion<br>¼ avocado<br>1 tbsp dressing (your preference)<br>Nutrition:<br>352kcal<br>20.1g total carbohydrates<br>33.8g protein<br>16.2g total fats |

The nutritional values have been calculated using the mobile application Lose It!™

## What We Know About Vegetarian Diets

### *Studies on the Vegetarian Diet*

A 2005 qualitative study by scholars Nick Fox and Katie Ward provides some insight into the reasons why people become vegetarian, investigating their motivations of people for doing so. The study, which included a forum that allowed the scholars to collect personal accounts as data, found that health and environmental concerns were the two main motivations for people choosing to follow a vegetarian diet.

Furthermore, they discovered a certain pattern among the participants of their study. Fox and Ward saw that, for most vegetarians, their initial motivation for following a vegetarian diet was to live a healthier lifestyle and improve their well-being. The scholars eventually found a trajectory of progress among the vegetarian participants — they saw that after initially becoming concerned with their health, vegetarians became concerned with the environment and the types of foods they were eating, and so they started. consuming ethically produced and organic foods. The idea of a "trajectory" within vegetarianism, a path to a more conscious way of life, is revealed by this study through the accounts and stories shared by vegetarian participants.

One participant named "Mark" spoke about the relationship between his health and his diet. Mark has experienced the physical benefits of following a total vegetarian (or vegan) diet; while he said that he does not call himself "vegan" or "vegetarian", he strictly follows a diet of solely plant, grains, and legumes due to the improvement of his physical and emotional well-being. Mark has found that when following a vegan diet, his "symptoms go away" and he feels "great" (Fox and Ward, 2005, p. 8).

Another account is a story shared by a participant "Vinny", who speaks about his health and history with food. For Vinny, the transition from his previous diet to a vegetarian diet involved a great improvement in his health. Vinny shares that, as a kid, he was overweight due to his diet of junk food — his diet excluded still water and vegetables as he only drank sugary soda drinks. The shift to a whole food and vegetarian diet was a challenge for Vinny because of his mental state, as well as defaulting to his previous eating habitats, but he eventually began to follow a vegetarian diet filled with fibre, grains, and legumes.

Similar to Vinny's story, a woman named "Lucy" was motivated to change to a vegetarian diet by many health issues, specifically her predisposition to certain genetic disorders carried in her family. Lucy decided to follow a vegetarian diet in order to prevent high cholesterol levels, as well as potential breast and ovarian cancer; for Lucy, the combination of exercise and following a vegetarian diet was her way of preventing herself from acquiring these illnesses.

Fox and Ward also discovered that sometimes, specific triggers can cause or motivate a person to change to a vegetarian diet. The story told by a woman named "Jane" explains how one specific experience changed her outlook on animal consumption. Jane shared her experience that occurred in her 7th grade science class, in which she took part in a practical exam which involved dissecting a chicken. Jane's perspective automatically shifted due to what she had observed during the event — Jane realized that the chicken's anatomy had similarities to a human's. After the experience, Jane started to follow a vegan diet, due to her strong belief in animal rights.

While Jane's reason for following a vegan diet is the protection of animals, "Bryn" decided to follow a vegetarian diet to protect humans as well. Bryn believes that non-organic animal farming — farming practices involving antibiotics within the popular mass-production of animal products — only increases the risk of antibiotic-resistant bacteria and dangerous viruses that could spread to humans. Bryn instead aims to consume organic dairy and eggs as a step to preventing disease outbreaks, while also not supporting the ill-treatment of animals.

This study, through observing the stories shared by participants, revealed how vegetarianism is an ever-changing and explorative journey. One's diet and lifestyle do not have to be set in stone, and we can learn and grow through educating ourselves and experiences in life. This work shared by Fox and Ward also highlights how vegetarianism varies, and how no matter what your motivation is, you can still live an intentional life by following a diet and making choices that work for you.

## FAQ: The Vegetarian Diet Explained

### Can I still eat gummy candies on a vegetarian diet?

The vegetarian diet is a diet that excludes meat, seafood, and poultry. Gummy sweets are not actual meat, but they often consist of gelatin, which is a binding agent made up of compacted animal tissue. Some vegetarians do eat gummy candies, while others do not — it is up to you to decide what is best for your body and lifestyle. Finding gelatin-free or vegetarian gummy candies has become an easier task than ever, as there are now many food brands that use plant-based binding agents in their products.

**Will I ever be able to eat meat again after being on a vegetarian diet for over 1 year?**

Never say never. There have been many stories of people who were total vegetarians for years, and then had to go back to eating animal products and seafood and poultry for health or personal reasons. It is never too late to adjust your diet— you need to listen to your body and monitor what diet works for your unique nutritional needs.

**Is it better to follow a plant-based or a vegetarian diet?**

No one diet is a perfect diet. If you are struggling to decide on which diet to start, you can observe your food preferences and nutritional needs, as well as your lifestyle choices. You could always trial both diets and see which one of the two works best for you, if one at all.

**Why are vegetarian diets still not promoted and followed in many societies?**

In most societies today and throughout history, human beings have been consuming meat. Our nutritional needs, our digestive system, and even our teeth are all made to consume meat — therefore, our response of following vegetarian diets to the livestock industry's actions goes against what human beings are naturally made to do. We also have to be aware of the other activities our ancestors did that we do not do today. We do not hunt for meat in our local land, as we have the con-venience of buying different types and cuts of meat whenever we feel like it. Vegetarianism is not universal because humans have grown accustomed to eating meat, and the livestock industry is gaining profit off this demand.

## Chapter Summary: The Vegetarian Diet Explained

This chapter was dedicated to defining the vegetarian diet and its varieties, and the many avenues one can go about following a diet that consists of fewer animal products. We looked at different meal options for each variety, giving an idea of the differences between these diets as an example so you can try them yourself. We then looked at how the vegetarian diet has been discussed and studied among the general public and the academic sphere. The study on the various motivations to follow a vegetarian diet by Fox and Ward gave us insight into the journeys of different people who are vegetarians, and the opinions and behaviors they hold.

Some lessons we learned from this chapter:

- The vegetarian diet is an umbrella term for various diets that include more plant-based products than animal products, including the total vegetarian diet (excludes all animal products), the lacto-ovo vegetarian diet (includes dairy and eggs), the lacto-vegetarian (includes dairy), the ovo-vegetarian diet (includes eggs), and the partial vegetarian diet (includes poultry or seafood occasionally).

- The vegetarian diet is a diverse diet, including processed and whole plant-based or animal-based products, and even animal meats on rare occasions.

- Many people follow a vegetarian diet because of health and animal welfare, or for environmental reasons.

# CHAPTER 5

# THE VEGETARIAN DIET AND YOUR HEALTH

## The Effects of the Vegetarian Diet on Your Health Explained

The vegetarian diet involves the exclusion of meat and other certain animal products. What does this shift or change do to our bodies? Does the lack of meat lead to a lack or deficiency in one's overall diet? Can and should a human being live a healthy and balanced life without meat? We often see that people ask about the issue or lack of protein concerning a diet that omits animal protein. As such, we need to investigate to find out what the effects of the vegetarian diet are on one's health, and if there are, in fact, protein deficiencies or decreases in energy.

Not only do we need to focus on physical health, but we also need to be aware of our emotional and psychological health, and of how one's diet could influence the way they feel as well as how their brain functions. Scientists have observed the effects of the diet on general health and nutrition in humans who follow an informed and balanced vegetarian diet plan. A 2006 study done by researchers Timothy J. Key,

Paul N. Appleby and Magdalena S. Rosell at Oxford University focused on the health effects of vegetarian and vegan diets., taking into account how education, culture, and genetics play a role in the outcomes of their study on vegetarianism. From their extensive research, Key Appleby, and Rosell found that the vegetarian diet is rich in nutrients while also low in others (Key, Appleby, and Rosell, 2006, p. 35). The vegetarian diet is rich in:

- Carbohydrates

- Dietary fiber

- N-6 fatty acids

- Folic acids

- Carotenoids

- Vitamins C and E

- Magnesium

Although these are vital nutrients, the vegetarian diet is low in certain other nutrients (Key, Appleby and Rosell, 2006, p. 35). The nutrients which the vegetarian diet is lower in are:

- Protein

- Saturated fat

- Long-chain N-3 fatty acids

- Retinol

- Vitamin B12

- Zinc

- Calcium (total vegetarian/vegan)

There is a general pattern and there are similar health effects shared by people who follow vegetarian diets. We need to remember and understand that all bodies are different and adjust our diets to fulfill our nutritional needs. For example, referring to these nutritional observations, we can assume that a person who does incorporate meat into their diet has higher amounts of saturated fats.

According to this study, the general consensus is that vegetarian diets have an impact on a person's physical body compared to diets that include meat. The most common physical health impacts and differences when following a vegetarian diet versus an omnivorous diet are: a lower BMI, lower plasma cholesterol concentration, and higher plasma homocysteine concentration. Although there are nutritional differences between vegetarian and non-vegetarian diets, experts believe that a *well-planned* and nutritionally conscious vegetarian diet can be beneficial to one's physical health. The American Dietetic Association and Dietitians of Canada, after observation and research, have stated that a vegetarian diet is an adequate diet for all stages of human life, including infancy, childhood, adolescence, and adulthood.

We do know that the differences between vegetarian and non-vegetarian diets cause nutritional differences, and we may often wonder how these nutritional differences affect health in the long-run. These nutritional differences affect our bodies, in both negative ways and in positive ones. Research suggests that these nutritional changes like high intake of dietary fiber, folic acid, vitamins C and E, and magnesium, as well as low intake of saturated fat, have potential health benefits.

### The Health Benefits of Following a Vegetarian Diet

- Lower risk of heart disease

- Low body mass index (BMI)
- Low cholesterol levels
- Low glucose levels
- Low risk of obesity
- Lower blood pressure
- Lower risk of colon cancer

### *The Health Risks of Following a Vegetarian Diet*

- Low BMI
- B12 Deficiency
- Zinc Deficiency
- Iron Deficiency (Heme Iron)
- Potential Anemia
- Potential Macrocytosis

## A Case Study: The Vegetarian Diet and Your Health

A study performed by researcher Roman Pawlak looked at whether vegetarian diets could be forms of prevention and management of diabetes. Pawlak's study was published in the Diabetes Spectrum, run by the American Diabetes Association (ADA) in 2017. Pawlak's work is in conversation and response to the many previous studies on the correlation between a vegetarian diet and the lower prevalence of type 2 diabetes. For Pawlak, this phenomenon is due to several consequences of following a vegetarian BAN diet, including improved or healthier weight, higher dietary fiber intake, and the absence of animal protein and animal-derived iron, or heme iron. These are the main contributors to why vegetarian— healthy total vegetarian diets in particular — have been viewed as effective forms of "treatment" to control glycemic levels and diabetes. This potential way of treating or alleviating diabetes is said to be due to the fact that vegetarian diets control plasma glucose much more effectively than other diets, even the low-carbohydrate diets that are commonly recommended to diabetes patients. Other findings inspired by Pawlak's work is the scientific knowledge that vegetarian diets are linked to weight reduction, improved serum lipid profile, and lower blood pressure; the idea that vegetarian diets can be used to prevent type 2 diabetes as well as improve blood glucose levels and management is central to Pawlak's study.

The study investigated the impact that brown-rice consumption, when on a vegan diet, would make on the glycemic control of 46 Korean diabetes patients versus the 47 control patients over the course of 12 weeks. The results of the study showed lower A1C levels (blood sugar levels) in both the control and the vegan diet group, but the latter showed more improvement — the stricter the compliance to a brown rice-incorporated vegan diet, the more significant the changes were in the patient's blood sugar levels (Pawlak, 2017). This is due to two factors: that the patients changed to a total vegetarian diet, and that they consumed slow-digesting complex carbohydrates like brown rice instead of white rice, which is a refined carbohydrate that spikes blood sugar levels.

This case study, one of many discussed in Pawlak's study, not only shows the significant health changes caused by following a vegetarian diet, but also the importance of food quality and nutritional knowledge. The vegetarian diet has many health benefits, but these benefits can only be seen if one follows a healthy and balanced diet. One can follow a vegetarian diet that includes processed potato chips, candy, high-fat foods like deep-fried carbs, or refined sugary foods like donuts — this diet is indeed vegetarian as it excludes animal meat, but it still includes high fat and sugar, as well as refined carbohydrates. It is not only about what you take out of your diet, but also what you put in it. If you exclude meat from your diet, what are you replacing those protein and caloric needs with? We need to remain educated and conscious of what we consume, how we consume it, and how it affects our well-being and overall health.

Another study discussed by Pawlak was the case of researcher Barsotti and colleagues, who investigated the diets of Buddhist monks in Thailand. The study involved two groups of participants, with the first group consisting of 25 vegan Buddhist monks, while the second group served as a control group of 25 non-vegetarians. Both groups were assessed in order to make a comparison between the health effects of the two diets. All participants underwent health checks, including renal function and overall health, in order to assess urinary proteins and the risk of cardiovascular disease. The results revealed that there was a significant difference concerning urinary protein among the two groups — the vegan group's average urinary protein was 1.4 mg/dL, while the non-vegetarian group's average was 5.2 mg/dL (Pawlak, 2017). This difference in urinary protein among the two groups reveals the improvement of kidney function as a result of following a vegan diet. This study not only provides scientific data about the health benefits of a total vegetarian diet, but it also sheds light on the cultural aspects of varying diets. Although this study was fully controlled and formalized, it also involved Buddhist monks who followed a vegetarian diet due to cultural and religious reasons, yet the outcome of their practices was also linked to their health. This shows us that a vegetarian diet and its health benefits can be experienced outside of Western science or formalized bio-medical studies. These monks have experienced the spiritual and physical benefits of following a vegetarian diet over generations. We can now see the vast and undiscovered benefits of the vegetarian diet, yet there is still much to uncover when it comes to its overall health effects.

## FAQ: The Vegetarian Diet and Your Health

### Will following a vegetarian diet make me lose fat?

You can lose fat by reducing your calories in addition to exercising and building muscle. Following a vegetarian diet can aid in your weight loss journey if you remain aware of the quantity and quality of foods you are consuming. As a vegetarian diet does reduce your animal fat intake, you might notice some changes in the way you look and feel, so you need to remember to find plant-based sources of protein to aid in fat loss and muscle growth. You can also speak to a dietician about your unique body and body goals.

### Is a lacto-vegetarian diet worse for my health than a total vegetarian diet?

This depends on your body's unique needs. As we read, the lacto-vegetarian diet does include animal fat, which can contribute to higher levels of cholesterol and inflammation in your body. In contrast, the total vegetarian diet excludes animal products, which can alter the necessary micronutrients needed to digest plant sources. Digestive issues can be experienced in both diets — if you are lactose intolerant, the lacto-vegetarian diet might disrupt your digestion, and if you struggle with a sensitive gut, then the excess fiber in a total vegetarian diet could also cause worsened gut issues. Your choice in a diet depends on your current health and physical experiences. Observe and learn about your body and your nutrition to know what diet will be most beneficial for your body and overall well-being.

**Will eating egg yolks increase my cholesterol?**

Egg yolks do have a certain amount of cholesterol in them, but excluding these will also lead to you not getting the nutrients that are in the yolk. Eggs are packed with beneficial and natural macronutrients and micronutrients. If you want to decrease your cholesterol levels, try to manage your animal fat intake and how you prepare your food. There is no need for you to cut eggs out of your diet. You can always aim to eat free-range eggs in moderation, instead of eating fried eggs for every meal.

**Does dairy yogurt really help the digestive system?**

Dairy yogurt includes natural healthy and extremely beneficial bacteria that is needed in the gut to aid in digestion. If your gut has a healthy microbiome, it will do its job better. Try to consume various probiotics like yogurt and kefir, or even fermented foods in order to provide your gut with a diverse range of bacteria.

## Chapter Summary: The Vegetarian Diet and Your Health

In this chapter, we learned how a vegetarian diet can affect your health. We explored how following the diet can have a positive or negative impact on your well-being — while this particular diet can improve your health by reducing unhealthy fats, cholesterol, blood pressure, and even the risk of certain cancers, we still need to be aware of the importance of balance. We learned how the vegetarian diet can be used as a form of treatment for diabetes type 1 and 2 through the study discussed by Roman Pawlak. The vegetarian diet, due to its diversity, can be adjusted for different health reasons.

Some lessons we learned from this chapter:

- You should take daily supplements for micronutrients that you cannot get from a vegetarian diet, such as vitamin B-12 and Omega-3, in addition to attending regular health and nutrition check-ups at your local general practitioner or dietitian.

- The vegetarian diet can be a form of treatment for type 1 and type 2 diabetes.

- Following a balanced and nutritionally adequate vegetarian diet can aid in your weight loss journey.

# CHAPTER 6

# THE VEGETARIAN DIET AND THE ENVIRONMENT

## The Effects of a Vegetarian Diet on the Environment Explained

When people follow a vegetarian diet, it is either for health or environmental reasons. Many people do not believe in the consumption of meat for either ethical or religious reasons. The consumption of meat affects the animals on our planet in more ways than one — although we know that there are unethical and abusive ways people farm animals, there are also other unethical practices involved in meat production and animal farming. The production of meat is aimed at making a profit, with high demand leading to an increase in competition. This reality of mass production and profitable animal farming leads to many farming practices that are dangerous to our environment.

This is especially true when it comes to the production of cow products. The environmental effects of a non-vegetarian diet are far greater than a vegetarian diet, and one very distinct difference is the issue of beef. In their study, Marlow, Hayes, Soret, Carter, Schwab, and Sabaté investigate the differences between the environmental effects of a vegetarian diet and the environmental effects of a non-vegetarian diet. The researchers looked at 6 environmental factors associated with the two diets, eventually deciding on the following list (Marlow et al., 2009).

1. Water resources

2. Energy consumption

3. Chemical fertilization

4. Pesticide use

5. Wastage

6. Land degradation

When it comes to water resources, in the United States there is a difference between the water usage for crops versus livestock. For cropland, most water needed is provided by rain, while agricultural production — including the irrigation of cropland and water for livestock — requires 80% of the water consumed in the country (Marlow et al., 2009).

Energy consumption in agricultural production varies depending on what is being produced. Technological advancements and use of fossil fuels has only encouraged the mass demand for products, even when they are out of season. This convenience requires more energy involved in the production and farming systems of produce, as well as in its transport. Due to the high demand for non-renewable fossil fuels, the supply is decreasing and will continue to decrease, meaning that the use of energy in agricultural production will need to be changed dramatically if to sustain the Earth.

The use of chemical fertilization has also increased in the United States; some chemicals, such as nitrogen fertilizer, are produced from non-renewable resources like petroleum. The use of fertilizers is important for modern-day crop farming, and the more we farm, the more fertilizer is needed. The results of overuse of fertilization include surface and groundwater contamination, air pollution, and a decrease in biodiversity.

The reliance on pesticides in farming has also increased worldwide, owing to unrestricted usage of pesticides caused by monoculture, cost-effectiveness, and the neglect of environmental and social cost of pesticides. Pesticides not only affect the environment, but also affect people's health — these pesticides can cause endocrine problems, immune dysfunction, neurological disorders, and cancers.

The increase in waste and pollution have been linked to animal production. As animal farming increases, so does animal waste, which leads to water, soil, and air pollution. The gases produced by livestock, such as carbon dioxide, methane, and nitrous oxide, have contributed to significant global issues like climate change. In the United States, the waste of 7 billion livestock is 130 times more than what is produced by 300 million humans (Marlow et al., 2009). These numbers are increasingly relevant as humans consume more livestock than needed. One human can eat chicken more than once a week, even more than once a day — think about how many chicken eggs people eat for breakfast, or add into recipes for baking?

The degradation of land is evident in the agriculture industry, as natural pastures are removed for livestock or the soil is eroded away by cropland pesticides. Despite all this, the livestock industry is the largest user of land — around 70% of all agricultural land has been used for livestock farming, which equates to 30% of the planet's land (Marlow et al., 2009). The increase in livestock production has caused several environmental issues relating to land. Some of the unfortunate consequences of livestock farming on land include the destruction of necessary and natural ecosystems, deforestation, destruction of biodiversity, desertification, compaction and erosion of soil, and the sedimentation of waterways, wetlands, and coastal areas. There has also been a link between invasive plants, animals, and organisms and the livestock industry. An example is zoonotic diseases like those seen in the poultry industry, where harmful avian influenza has been transferred among livestock and then to other animals, including humans.

### *The Positive Environmental Effects of a Vegetarian Diet*

- Less greenhouse gas emissions
- Less fossil fuels used for energy
- More available and healthier land for biodiversity
- A decrease in the risk of zoonotic diseases
- A decrease in air, water, and soil pollution

### *The Negative Environmental Effects of a Vegetarian Diet*

- Land and soil erosion
- Destruction of biodiversity
- Deforestation
- Potential poisoning of soil, water, plants, and animals

# A Case Study: The Vegetarian Diet and the Environment

Researchers Linda Bacon and Dario Krpan investigated the effects a vegetarian designed restaurant menu would have on diners in a 2018 study. Following in the footsteps of previous research done on restaurant menu design, Bacon and Krpan wanted to see if adjusting a restaurant menu to a vegetarian one would influence people's choice to choose a more ethical meal instead of a standard omnivorous meal. The researchers were also aware of the fact that people's past behaviors can also influence their choices, and that this is the same when it comes to their food choices.

Bacon and Krpan wanted to use these phenomena in their study on vegetarian meals. The researchers wanted to know whether the people who claimed to eat more vegetarian meals in the week would be more influenced to order a vegetarian meal off of a restaurant menu. They were also focused on the positive environmental implications of regularly eating vegetarian food, and whether this factor would steer the participants into a more pro-vegetarian diet.

The study went as follows. Participants were asked about their meals for the past week, then randomly assigned to four different restaurant menus. These four menus were:

1. The control menu — all meals were presented in the same way.

2. The recommendation menu — the vegetarian meal was the chef's recommended meal on the menu.

3. The descriptive menu — a menu that included a description of a vegetarian menu that made it appear more appealing.

4. The vegetarian menu — a menu with a separate vegetarian section.

At the end of the study, the results were not what the researchers expected. The recommendation menu and the descriptive menu increased the chances of the participants choosing a vegetarian meal among those who were not regular vegetarian food eaters. Surprisingly, the vegetarian menu did not influence the choices of the participants, regardless of whether or not they were regular vegetarian eaters. Therefore, Bacon and Krpan advised businesses and other researchers to be conscious of people's past food behaviors, and to aim at adjusting and personalizing meals in order to encourage people to choose and follow a more sustainable diet. People do not want to be forced into making the "right" choice; they want to feel in control of their decisions, while also helping the environment on their own terms. This study is a really important one, showcasing how people enjoy variety and freedom of choice despite the very real and serious environmental effects the consumption of animal products has on the environment. We need to think of creative and unique ways of encouraging and inspiring people to make daily choices that work to protect the environment, and not add to the current environmental issues we face today.

## FAQ: The Vegetarian Diet and the Environment

### Is it ethical to eat eggs?

The answer is not straightforward. Many people buy eggs as it is a staple in their diet, including a vegetarian diet. We do know that hens lay eggs naturally and do not need to be forced or exploited to do this, but we also know that people *have* exploited hens in their ability to provide a great natural protein for us. The unethical side rarely seen in regards to chicken eggs are the practices involved in battery farming, where chickens live in tiny cages and are pumped with hormones to lay as many eggs as possible for human consumption. To avoid supporting battery farming, you can buy eggs at your local market from local farmers who raise free-range chickens. You can also look for eggs that have "free-range" or "happy chickens" stamped on them, or labeled on their packaging.

**Is the dairy industry worse for the environment than the meat industry?**

If we look at it as the same industry collectively, then it will reveal how the mass production of cow and sheep products is a larger contributing factor to the negative impacts on the environment. Think about how much milk you drink daily — you add milk to your coffee, your cereal, and as a drink with your meals. Do you eat a steak for every meal of the day? We need to stop comparing the meat industry and dairy industry, and instead see these two as one big industry. We have learned that the farming of cows, for either meat or dairy, places a large threat on our environment. The best way to reduce your carbon footprint and protect the environment is to reduce the number of animal products you consume; whether you are drinking milk or eating a beef burger, both increase the demand for cow farming.

**How do I know if my vegetarian products are made ethically?**

You can look for labels and logos that say "vegan", "cruelty-free", "sustainably sourced", or "ethical". You can also make regular shopping trips to local farmer's markets.

## Will not eating meat protect me from animal-borne bacteria and viruses?

By not supporting the livestock industry, you will reduce the demand and the possibility of zoonotic diseases. You need to remember that there are many animal-borne diseases, and other people who are exposed to these diseases can still pass these on to you despite your efforts to avoid eating meat. You should try to be cautious of people and keep up your hygiene practices, so wash your hands regularly when around people, or before and after meals. You should also avoid people who are showing symptoms of flu, while regularly reading the news and keeping updated on health and safety warnings.

## Chapter Summary: The Vegetarian Diet and the Environment

This particular chapter discussed the ways the vegetarian diet can affect the environment. We looked at how the vegetarian diet compares to an omnivorous diet when it comes to negative environmental effects — although both the vegetarian diet and omnivorous diet have several environmental implications, the vegetarian diet does not threaten the environment as much as the omnivorous diet due to the drastic harm done by the livestock industry. Adopting a vegetarian diet is a good step towards lowering your carbon footprint. An interesting study we looked at was performed by Bacon and Krpan, who investigated one way of reducing our carbon footprint through the promotion of vegetarian food. While the vegetarian diet is gaining increased popularity and support, there is still more work that needs to be done, and more energy, time, and money allocated for the diet to become a universal lifestyle.

Some lessons we learned in this chapter:

- The vegetarian diet can still contribute to environmental issues like soil and land erosion, as well as the destruction of natural ecosystems and biodiversity.

- It is easier for people to follow a vegetarian diet if they are reminded of environmental issues and if they have a strong conviction to lower their carbon footprint on a daily basis.

- Reducing the demand and supply of meat can prevent and reduce the rates at which zoonotic diseases are created and transferred among different animals, including humans.

# CHAPTER 7

# THE VEGAN DIET EXPLAINED

## What is a Vegan Diet?

### Defining a Vegan Diet

The vegan diet is defined as a diet that excludes all meats and animal-produced substances. These products include meat, poultry and seafood, dairy, eggs, gelatin, and even honey. Vegans also avoid eating other processed or packaged products if they have ingredients or traces of animal produced substances such as milk or skim milk powder, whey powder, chicken broth, and binding and glossing agents, including wax or tissue/fat of living creatures. There is a difference between the vegan diet and "vegan". The vegan diet refers to food, but oftentimes does heavily impact one's shopping and consumption of products, whereas "vegan" also involves the exclusion of any animal produced substances, centering around inedible items, such as clothes or cosmetics and other household products.

The vegan diet has become increasingly popular in the last decade. While there has also been increased behavior by which people seek to incorporate organic, free-range, and sustainably sourced animal products in their diets, the vegan diet is still more popular than ever before. This social phenomenon is due to the demand for and accessibility of vegan food and products, as well as having more access to information about the cruel and harsh conditions and treatment occurring in the global animal production industry. Another reason for the growth of vegan diets is the ever-expanding and evident global issue of climate change, which research has shown to be caused and exacerbated by the animal production industry through actions such as cow farming.

As such, the vegan diet has been deemed by several recent studies as a significant potential path to the Earth's recovery, as well as an antidote to increasing global obesity and type 2 diabetes rates. The vegan diet, similar to the vegetarian and plant-based diets, is associated with the same motivations to follow it, referring to mainly health and environmental reasons. Unlike the vegetarian and plant-based diets, however, the vegan diet is much more focused on ethics and morality. People often choose to go vegan due to their awareness of the current unethical animal farming industries. Other issues like the use of antibiotics and growth hormones in animal production, as well as potential animal-borne diseases stemming from the practices and conditions of animal produce farms, are reasons for why many people adopt a vegan diet. Vegans are often much more conscious of where and how their food is produced — a vegan diet does not include any product from a living and breathing creature, as it is seen as unethical and unjust to exploit and often mistreat a living creature.

While we can see that the vegan diet has exploded in popularity and may be a great opportunity to transform your life, we also need to understand that it is much less popular than other diets. This is because it has been more difficult or inconvenient for people to follow a vegan diet, the reasons for which include cultural norms, nutritional misinformation or misconceptions, inaccessibility, cost, peer pressure, health, and diet conditions. One example of misinformation around nutrition is the idea that milk gives you strong bones, while most research suggests that a vegan diet, if implemented properly, is adequate for this goal because it is high in other nutrients that are beneficial for bone health. We were told as children that the consumption of cow's milk is necessary to grow big and strong. As we study and learn more, the truth reveals itself and we have to sometimes unlearn what we grew up believing. Human bodies, both after infancy and as they age, actually produce less lactase, the enzyme that helps us digest the lactose found in milk. This is because humans do not need to drink animal milk, or their mother's milk, after a certain age. For researcher Robert D. McCracken, this lack of or reduction of lactase in the human body is viewed as an example of "dietary evolution" (McCracken, 1971). The decrease or deficiency in lactase leads to the difficulty or inability to digest milk and reap the apparent nutritional rewards animal milk has to offer. With this perspective, many vegans and even non-dairy consumers believe that humans were never meant to consume the milk of other animals.

Although a vegan diet is and does seem restrictive and quite limited in what you can eat, in reviewing our studies and observations alongside the convenience of new forms of trade and farming, we have a new-found wide variety of vegan foods that are delicious and satiating as well as nutritious. Due to the vegan diet gaining popularity, there are more nutritional plant sources than ever before; we have discovered just how diverse and beneficial plants and grains can be for the human body.

## *Vegan Meal Ideas*

Disclaimer: These meals can be tried and implemented in a vegan diet that also includes a vitamin B-12 supplement. You should not follow a vegan diet that does not include animal products without supplementing the B-12 vitamin daily.

Here are some examples of vegan meals:

| Meal | Ingredients |
| --- | --- |
| **Breakfast** | Smoothie Bowl:<br><br>2 frozen bananas<br><br>1 tbsp nut butter (your preference)<br><br>1 heaped scoop plant protein powder<br><br>1 tsp cocoa<br><br>1 tbsp cacao nibs<br><br>¼ mixed nuts<br><br>Nutrition:<br><br>725kcal<br><br>69.9g total carbohydrates<br><br>35.7g protein<br><br>31.1g total fats |

| | |
|---|---|
| **Lunch** | Tofu Scramble:<br>1 cup mashed tofu<br>½ cherry tomatoes<br>½ spinach<br>¼ sliced bell peppers<br>¼ sliced onion<br>1 tsp paprika<br>1 slice bread (your preference)<br>Nutrition:<br>228kcal<br>26.2g total carbohydrates<br>17.6g protein<br>7.9g total fats |
| **Dinner** | Lentil Salad:<br>1 cup cooked lentils<br>½ cherry tomatoes<br>½ cup cubed cucumber<br>¼ grated carrot<br>¼ cup cooked beetroot<br>¼ avocado<br>1 tbsp nutritional yeast flakes<br>1 tbsp pumpkin seeds<br>1 tbsp balsamic vinegar<br>1 tbsp extra virgin olive oil<br>Nutrition:<br>478kcal<br>61.6g total carbohydrates<br>25g protein<br>29.9g total fats |

The nutritional values were calculated by the mobile application Lose It!™

## What We Know About Vegan Diets

### *Studies on the Vegan Diet*

A study performed by Pamela Kerschke-Risch in Germany on the popularity of veganism in the country was published in the city of Hamburg in 2015. The study centers around the results of online surveys done as part of a German quantitative sociological study — this study focuses particularly on *people*, and how their behaviors and opinions can be interpreted to better understand the growth and reality of vegan diets in the country.

One particular survey performed from July to August 2013 was an anonymous online survey, which involved 852 vegans answering a specific set of questions about the motives for following this particular diet, as well as the current national situation of the diet. After much investigation and interpretation of the survey answers, the findings illustrated by Kerschke-Risch revealed that there are three main motives for following a vegan diet: the reports on factory farming, the protection of the climate, and health. These findings are very similar to the findings of the study done 10 years earlier by Fox and Ward on motivations for following a vegetarian diet (Kerschke-Risch 2015, p.98).

In addition to the motives of vegan's choices in following a vegan diet, other aspects of this study revealed results that created a clearer picture of the social phenomenon. These additional factors included participants 'age and gender, the duration of vegan dietary behavior, the approach to a vegan diet, and the assessment of the difficulties of a vegan diet. The results of these aspects describe the population of the study, providing further insight into the attitudes and behaviors of vegans in Germany. Kerschke-Risch discovered that, similar to previous studies on vegetarians, women made up the majority of the vegan population, making up 80% of the vegans who were involved in the particular study. The average age of the population was 30-34 (Kerschke-Risch, 2015, p. 99).

The duration of practicing the vegan diet amongst the population was also quite short, with most people having only followed the diet for 2 to 5 years. Only 12% of the population had claimed to be experienced "long-term vegans" (Kerschke-Risch, 2015, p.99). The general approach to starting a vegan diet was also clear, as many people described an intermediate phase in their diet where they would first begin to cut out meat for a period of time, before eventually transitioning to a diet that excluded animal products — this "intermediate stage" was followed by more than 73% of vegans studied (2015, p.100). Allowing their body to adjust to a diet without meat before making more extreme and challenging dietary changes enabled the participants to test the diet in a way that worked with their particular body and lifestyle.

Furthermore, the results of the motives and the participants' assessments on the difficulty of a vegan diet were also discussed by Kerschke-Risch. The most popular motivator in participants 'choice to start a vegan diet were educational reports on factory farming that revealed the unethical farming practices, the mistreatment of animals, and the environmental dangers involved in the production of livestock. The least important motivator was found to be the food scandals around animal products. Interestingly, there were more women than men influenced by specific examples of food scandals and farming practices (Kerschke-Risch, 2015). This could be because of the fact women made up the majority of the vegan population in this study. The last factor discussed by Kerschke-Risch was the idea of the vegan diet being difficult to follow. Like most in this study, there is a general and popular answer when asking whether the vegan diet is easier to follow today: "yes, definitely" (Kerschke-Risch, 2015, p.100).

Kerschke-Risch's study also revealed other patterns among the attitudes of vegans. One popular opinion in Germany is that it has become easier for people to follow a vegan diet in recent years. Due to the increase in the accessibility of vegan products, there has been a boom in vegan production. More than a third of the people participating in the survey had been vegan for two years or more (Kerschke-Risch, 2015, p.98).

## FAQ: The Vegan Diet Explained

**Is honey vegan or not?**

Technically, no. It is made by bees, making it a byproduct of a living creature that is often exploited as humans profit off its natural byproduct.

**Can I be vegan and still wear leather and wool?**

Yes, you can still follow a vegan diet and wear leather and wool. The vegan diet is different than the vegan lifestyle. You can follow a vegan diet alone, although limiting your purchases on all animal products and not just edible ones is the most effective way to live a lifestyle that is beneficial for the environment.

**How do I know if processed and packaged snacks from the grocery store are really vegan?**

You can look at the front or back of packaged goods and seek any certified sign or logo that includes a green heart or plant, or a checkmark. Some logos also include the words "vegan" or "cruelty-free". It is suggested you perform your own research and investigation into the brand or company to determine if their product is completely vegan.

**Do I have to cook all my meals to ensure my food is 100% vegan?**

No. In recent years, due to the increase in demand for vegan and plant-based goods, there are now many brands of frozen vegan meals and plant-protein snacks. You can search for them in the vegan aisle or vegan products section at your local grocery store.

## Chapter Summary: The Vegan Diet Explained

This chapter was an informative introduction to the vegan diet. We defined the diet and lifestyle and discussed the reasons why it is beneficial for people, other living creatures, and the planet. Although the vegan diet is the most restrictive diet among the three diets we have discussed, we explored the ways one can easily follow this diet, and examples of meals were provided. We considered a German study done by researcher Pamela Kerschke-Risch, which focused on the reasons behind one's choice to follow a vegan diet. We looked at how this diet is gaining popularity in the western world. This could be a promising sign of potential positive changes for the environment in the future.

Some lessons we learned in this chapter:

- Although the vegan diet seems more restrictive compared to the plant-based and vegetarian diets, it consists of diverse, plentiful and often unheard-of sources of nutrients, which are all provided by plants grown from the Earth.

- A great and versatile source of vegan protein is soy, which is found in products like tofu and plant-based milks and yogurt.

- Due to the increase in accessibility and economic means, many western societies have witnessed a growth in followers of the vegan diet and lifestyle.

# CHAPTER 8

# THE VEGAN DIET AND YOUR HEALTH

## The Effects of a Vegan Diet on Your Health Explained

The health effects of the vegan diet were studied and discussed by scholar Winstion J. Craig, who looked at the health consequences of following a vegan diet in a 2009 study. Craig acknowledges the health benefits of nutritional changes caused by most vegetarian diets, as these diets are high in many nutrients such as fiber, folic acid, vitamins C and E, potassium, and magnesium, as well as unsaturated phytochemicals and fats. Despite these nutritional effects being beneficial, and often also occurring in vegan diets, the difference between these two dietary paths is the presence of saturated fat. Craig notes that vegan diets have less saturated fats and cholesterol compared to vegetarian diets, likely due to the presence of animal products and fats incorporated into vegetarian diets — this has the potential to lead to more saturated fats and cholesterol levels from foods like fatty cheeses and yogurts, as well as cow's milk and eggs with egg yolks.

Although this could seem like a health benefit, due to the fact that saturated fats have been deemed as "unhealthy fats" and high cholesterol levels have been associated with higher risks of heart diseases, Craig states that there may be nutritional deficiencies caused by a vegan diet because it excludes some fats and nutrients only found in animal products. The issue is the lack of micronutrients usually found in a vegan diet; these micronutrients are vitamin B-12 and vitamin D, calcium, omega 3 fatty acids, iron, and zinc. Craig encourages vegans to seek supplements for these nutrients, due to the lack of these nutrients in plant sources and the limited bioavailability of iron and zinc in some plants. One can supplement these through vegan certified synthetic vitamin supplements, fortified cereals, and processed and packaged foods, such as vegan frozen food brands or vegan protein bars.

In Craig's study, the vegan diet is said to be higher in these nutrients (Craig, 2009):

- Dietary fiber
- Folic acid
- Vitamins C and E
- Magnesium
- Iron
- Phytochemicals

While the vegan diet does include many nutritional benefits sourced from plants and grains, it is lower in the following (Craig, 2009):

- Calories
- Saturated fat
- Long-chain N-3 fatty acids, such as Omega-3
- Cholesterol

- Vitamins D and B-12

- Zinc

- Calcium

Part of the way the body functions is determined by the things we eat, affecting the hormonal and digestive systems specifically. Therefore, the vegan diet does change the hormonal and digestive functioning of the body, which is directly connected to the change in amounts, availability, and digestibility of particular nutrients in the body. Due to the changes in hormones, and because our bodies are holistic beings, our physical body also affects our emotional body. Mentally, some people feel emotionally lighter or more energized when they do not consume animal products. Biologically, the body is digesting the food better — therefore, the nutrients in the food are being used, resulting in an increase in energy via calories and vitamins that correlate with how our body functions. If we are deficient in vitamin C, we will see the physical and then emotional effects of this. When a person does not get enough vitamin C from their diet because they are not eating enough citrus fruits and berries, they will feel lethargic, and will be more prone to the seasonal flu. This consequence could lead to a person becoming less productive and more isolated, further affecting their emotional and social well-being.

We need to treat our body as a complex machine, like a car. A car needs fuel in the form of food, as well as cleaning and services, and as it ages it causes the driver more problems. Our bodies and minds are much more complex than cars, but this analogy makes sense because we use our bodies every day. We need to be aware of what our body needs — every single body is unique and has different needs, different ailments, and different strengths and weaknesses. When you follow a certain diet, such as the vegan diet, you need to educate yourself, absorb the material, trial, and then observe and listen to your body, making changes where necessary. Due to the fact that the vegan diet is higher in fiber, some experience excess gas and bowel issues, so it's important to slowly introduce the diet and give the body time to adapt and adjust. Some people have to follow or cannot follow a vegan diet because of their pre-existing health conditions — this highlights the importance of education on your specific health needs prior to changing the way you eat.

### The Health Benefits of Following a Vegan Diet

- Lower risk of cardiovascular disease
- Low body mass index (BMI)
- Low cholesterol levels
- Low glucose levels
- Low risk of obesity
- Lower blood pressure
- Lower risk of colon cancer and other cancers
- Potentially lower risk of osteoporosis
- Potentially lower risk of type 2 diabetes

### The Health Risks of Following a Vegan Diet

- Low BMI
- B12 deficiency, which can lead to neurologic and psychiatric issues including dementia, disorientation, concentration difficulties, mood and motor difficulties, paresthesia, and psychoses

- Zinc deficiency

- Vitamin D deficiency

- Iron deficiency (Heme iron)

- Potential eye and brain dysfunction

- Potential anemia

- Potential Macrocytosis

- Indigestion, caused by excessive undigested fiber

## A Case Study: The Vegan Diet and Your Health

In 2020, scholars Daniel Davey, Shane Malone, and Brendan Egan studied the case of a Gaelic soccer player of 25 years old who followed a vegan diet. The man was young, an athlete, and needed many nutrients to sustain his active lifestyle. In addition, his physical performance and overall well-being were monitored. Due to the restrictive nature of the vegan diet and the high nutritional needs of an athlete, the study provides vital information in the general investigation of the potential health effects the diet has on the health of human bodies.

The study considered whether the transition from an omnivorous diet to a vegan diet would change the athlete's performance, energy levels, and overall nutrition. At the beginning of the study, the man's physical information was recorded. The man was 25 years old, his height was 6.2ft and his weight was 193.6lbs, with 161.5lbs of lean body mass and 11.3% body fat (Davey et al., 2020).

The man's dietary transition from an omnivorous diet to a vegan diet began at the start of the competitive season, so optimal training was needed. The study involved testing and observation of nutritional intake, body composition, and match-play running performance. With this assistance and nutritional knowledge, results showed that the athlete was receiving adequate nutrients from a vegan diet for his body and active lifestyle. His performance was identical to when he was consuming an omnivorous diet. In the study, he followed a provided meal plan that incorporated plant-based protein and protein powder, as well as fats from seeds — there was also an additional enhancement of a multivitamin supplement that was taken regularly, which included iron, iodine, calcium, vitamin B-12, and vitamin D. This study demonstrates that, although the vegan diet can be followed successfully with nutritional needs met in athletes, the transition from an omnivorous diet to a vegan diet and maintenance after the transition is an essential part to its success. One should not transition to a vegan diet and blindly cut out all animal products without regular medical checks, tests, and nutritional knowledge of their specific body and its needs. Knowing what nutrients your body needs to perform optimally, as well as knowing exactly how you are going to replace the essential nutrients in the products you cut out is important. Following these informative and eye-opening guidelines prevent potential health risks to your body.

## FAQ: The Vegan Diet and Your Health

### How do I know if my vegan diet is causing me to be deficient in certain nutrients?

You can get regular blood tests at your local health clinic or general practitioner. If you do find that you are deficient in certain vitamins, you should take a vegan multivitamin and receive a B-12 injection, in addition to a daily B-12 supplement. Speak to your doctor if you have any health concerns.

**Can I follow a vegan diet while I am pregnant?**

Yes. By following a balanced vegan diet it will provide most, if not all, of your macronutrients and micronutrients. Although iron and calcium are not as abundant on a vegan diet, you can take daily supplements to ensure you are getting enough micronutrients. A prenatal supplement is also vital during pregnancy.

**Will following a vegan diet cause me to have a more restrictive mindset when it comes to eating?**

If you have a history of restrictive eating, then try to seek help to unlearn the thought patterns before beginning your vegan diet. If you do start your vegan diet and find that you are experiencing feelings of guilt, which leads to obsessing over your food and inhibits you from living out your daily routines, then you should seek help from a medical professional. In doing so, you can get advice on how to move forward in your vegan journey, or if you should continue it.

**How do I gain weight on a vegan diet?**

If you are battling to gain weight on a vegan diet, try adding more healthy and high caloric fats to your diet. You can cook or drizzle your food in extra virgin olive oil or avocado oil, or top your meals with fatty seeds like chia, pumpkin, and sunflower seeds. You can also reduce foods that are high in quantity but low in caloric quality, like leafy greens and raw vegetables.

# Chapter Summary: The Vegan Diet and Your Health

In this chapter, we focused on the topics of health and nutrition of the vegan diet, discovering the many health effects associated with it — specifically, we looked at micronutrients like fatty acids, zinc, iron, and B-12 as vitamins that are not prevalent or not found in vegan foods and therefore need to be supplemented. The health benefits and risks are more or less of equal weight compared to other diets, however, the vegan diet is much more restrictive, and can pose a great threat to your health if not implemented thoroughly and wisely. Although there is a risk of forming deficiencies on a vegan diet, Davey, Malone, and Egan's case study of a professional athlete following the vegan diet proved that it is very much possible to perform optimally if one's health is regularly monitored and includes a balanced meal plan and supplements.

Some lessons we learned from this chapter:

- A vitamin B-12 supplement needs to be taken regularly with the vegan diet, as you cannot get this vitamin from natural vegan food and cannot rely on fortified foods like cereals and processed vegan products that add vitamins to their products.

- It's important to do research on nutrition and to be well-informed about the health and nutritional adjustments that need to be made before adopting a vegan diet.

- The vegan diet reduces inflammation, therefore lowering the risk of heart disease and diabetes due to lack of animal fat in the diet.

# CHAPTER 9

# THE VEGAN DIET AND THE ENVIRONMENT

## The Effects of a Vegan Diet on the Environment Explained

Although vegetarian and Chai, van der Voort, Grofelnik, Eliasdottir, Klöss, and Perez-Cueto diets have become popular in recent years due to health and environmental reasons, the vegan diet has been said to be the most beneficial for the planet. Chai lead a review in 2019 on vegan, vegetarian, and omnivorous diets, and found that the vegan diet is the most environmentally conscious and friendly out of all the diets, emitting the lowest levels of greenhouse gas emissions. Health and animal welfare have been the main motivations for those adopting a vegetarian or plant-based diet, however, due to the rapid increase of greenhouse gas emissions, and climate change becoming more and more evident, vegans have found a more effective way to reduce their carbon footprint.

The livestock industry has posed a great threat to our planet's well-being for many years, yet in recent years people have become more educated and more conscious of the environmental impact humans and production has and continues to have on our planet. The livestock industry requires a large percentage of our Earth's land, water, and fossil fuel energy. The massive amount of resources utilized harms the very source that has provided them. The modern farming industry has not been implementing sustainable farming systems, as greed has clouded our judgement; both consumers 'greed for more convenient produce and manufacturers 'greed for a bigger profit. It has become an unsustainable and threatening cycle. We can lessen the negative impacts on the environment and reduce the rate of climate change by reducing our carbon footprints, while also protecting our planet's natural ecosystems and biodiversity.

Although we can simply downsize our consumption of meat, which decreases both our carbon footprint and our water consumption, we still need to be conscious of the fact that the production of dairy also contributes to high amounts of greenhouse gas emissions. Decreasing the amount of dairy products consumed in combination with decreasing meat consumed is more environmentally friendly and more effective in decreasing our carbon footprint. The production of meat and dairy is estimated to contribute to 80% of greenhouse gas emissions in the food industry, while making up 24% of the world's overall greenhouse gas emissions (Chai et al., 2019, p.11). These greenhouse gas emissions seem to be more prevalent in the farming of livestock, specifically grazing animals like cows and sheep. Poultry and pig farming do not contribute to as many emissions, however, they still impact the environment. The farming of pigs and chickens pose other environmental hazards specifically to other animals and sometimes humans through the transmission of zoonotic diseases. We have seen throughout history how the farming of livestock has disrupted natural ecosystems, in addition to the well-being of human beings — examples such as mad cow disease, swine flu, and the more recent coronavirus strains have all caused pandemics.

Furthermore, the vegan lifestyle not only is responsible for the prevention and reduction of dangerous environmental effects, but also carries a philosophy with it. The majority of people who follow the vegan diet also adopt the vegan lifestyle which involves no consumption of any products that have been derived from an animal; for example: cosmetics, clothing, accessories, and furniture. Living with this philosophy in mind directly reduces one's carbon footprint on the planet by reducing the demand for animal-sourced products— for instance, if we do not buy leather shoes, we will be reducing the demand for leather, which is reliant on the farming of cows. If we do not buy wool, we will be reducing the demand for sheep farming, which also accounts for a large amount of greenhouse gas emissions.

As a result, vegans in both diet and lifestyle have opted for vegan products like vegan leather or faux fur. Many people, vegan or not, have gravitated towards certified vegan and cruelty-free cosmetics, as most of the products we use on our bodies have been tested on animals. Some cosmetic products have animal products in them such as wax or fatty tissue, which is often used as a binding agent. These practices are seen as unethical and harmful to all living things. Lab testing can bring about several dangerous and biological consequences. For these reasons, there has been an increase in demand for and supply of vegan, cruelty-free, and organic products. Staying informed of our everyday behaviors and choices, and beginning to ask questions about products in the market can help develop our consciousness of consumption. Was this product made locally, or is it imported? Does this product include animal products? Is this product a certified vegan and cruelty-free product by local and international authorities? Is this product's packaging recycled or recyclable?

The vegan diet and lifestyle bring awareness to the cost of modern-day human life; it reminds us that human beings can live a healthy and sustainable life by consuming natural produce and plants. It emphasizes the ideology of wanting or needing to live ethically and benefit the planet. The higher demand for vegan products is healthier for the environment than animal products. Although vegan foods tend to be more environmentally friendly, there are still manufacturing processes that can be harmful. If you want to follow a vegan diet, try to choose the oat milk that comes in a glass or recyclable bottle. Some almond milk brands are imported, however, you can choose to avoid them and drink local plant-based milks that have not been mass-produced, imported, and result in negative environmental effects. Try buying an organic and locally produced shampoo with plant-based ingredients, as opposed to the imported big brand shampoo that is unclear about its production process. Being vegan is best when one remains open and honest and is trying to change their lifestyle to benefit themself. When you know better, you can do better by doing *your* best.

### *The Positive Environmental Effects of Following a Vegan Diet*

- A significant reduction in greenhouse gases
- Lower levels of water waste
- Lower levels of air, water, and land pollution
- Lower risks of animal-borne diseases
- Less demand for ruminant dairy animals, like cows and sheep

*The Negative Environmental Effects of Following a Vegan Diet*

- Potential biodiversity reduction

- Land and soil erosion

- Non-recyclable and non-biodegradable waste

- Poisoning of plants, animals, water systems, and people

## A Case Study: The Vegan Diet and the Environment

A 2021 study by scholars Yeong-Hyeon Choi and Kyu-Hye Lee reveals the cycle of veganism and its strong link to environmentalism and consumers 'behaviors. Choi and Lee looked at the patterns and reasons behind the "ethical" consumer buying fake leather and fur, as well as the correlation between education and awareness around vegan materials and their impact on environmental change. The scholars acknowledge that there has been a rise in the demand for ethical production in many industries, specifically the food and fashion industries.

This particular study looked at the recent but evident global consumer transition. Due to the increase in accessible global news and information, people have become aware and more informed about how their products are made, leading to an increase in vegan materials. Despite their diet, people have been increasingly interested in vegan materials. The reasons behind this increase in interest and demand could be due to peer pressure, animal rights, the faster exchange of news, or for the ego boost people may experience for feeling like they are buying ethically. For Choi and Lee, the reasons behind the interest are in regards to the ethics that involve animals and the environment.

Choi and Lee studied consumers 'social media posts from 2018 to 2019, making use of search engine applications like Twitter and Google search tools. The scholars examined and followed the patterns of users 'language and behavior across this particular time period — initially, people spoke about animal materials and associated these materials with topics such as animal rights, animal abuse, and animal protection. From these topics, an interest in animal welfare was sparked, evolving into conversations about cruelty-free products like faux fur and vegan leather. In the last stages of behavior, the consumers were now more involved with these products and refer to their impacts on the environment and what "eco" or "eco-friendly" is defined as. From this multiple-month case study, there exists a connection between the products we consume and the environment. This is a single example of how an interest in the vegan lifestyle can snowball into discussions of other important topics and aspects of life. The study showcases that given there were more accessible and affordable vegan and cruelty-free products in our stores, the exposure would affect general public knowledge and consumption. The option to buy vegan products would slowly decrease the demand for animal production. The freedom of choice and the luxury of variety cause consumers to be invested when they're shopping. If consumers know that their products, luxury or not, are being made ethically and sustainably, it could lead to an emotional manifestation, cleansing the guilt of buying an unethical product.

Ultimately, if vegan products can make consumers feel happier while also protecting the environment, there should be more campaigns for vegan products. Unlike food, which holds a much more complex connection and relationship with the body, a designer handbag is external and can rest on both its looks and its reputation. If people have the opportunity to buy affordable quality vegan materials that protect the environment over materials that destroy the environment, they most likely would buy the former. These vegan purchases will make consumers more aware of the production process of goods, which can lead to them becoming interested in other unethical production practices. This study is an example of the possibilities of environmental recovery through creating a supply-and-demand chain for vegan materials.

## FAQ: The Vegan Diet and the Environment

### Is going vegan the best way to save the planet?

It is one of the best ways to save the planet, as it is the diet with the lowest carbon footprint. If you are able to consume ethically-sourced and manufactured vegan products it will be a great way to make your contribution to saving our planet.

### Are imported vegan products bad for the planet?

They are not as bad as imported animal products, but it is better to buy locally sourced vegan products to prevent the demand of fossil fuels used in transportation.

### Is the mass production of vegan products bad for the environment?

Yes, but not as bad as with animal production and farming. There have unfortunately been incidents like the almond industry in California or palm oil farming in the Amazon forest which have led to the destruction of indigenous plants, creatures, and ecosystems. Try to buy products that are certified as sustainably sourced and look at the packaging for the ingredients. Try to avoid buying vegan products that do not have ethically-grown palm oil in them.

**Are all vegan products good for the environment?**

No, as some vegan products may still be packed in non-recyclable packaging. Many vegan products might exclude animal products, but could still include non-biodegradable materials which could add to the global plastic pollution in our oceans. Awareness of the ingredients of your vegan products is great, but the awareness of the materials used in their packaging is even better. Vegan products that are packaged in plastic and are imported can still be harmful to the environment, despite not being associated with animal production. Try to look for vegan products that are locally sourced and have certified vegan, sustainably sourced, and cruelty-free logos on them.

## Chapter Summary: The Vegan Diet and the Environment

In this chapter, we discussed the many effects that the food industry has on the environment, coming to the conclusion that the vegan diet contributes to the least amount of greenhouse gas emissions, water wastage, and pollution of the three major diets considered. While this fact gives promise and hope for the future, there still exists other potentially dangerous factors in the manufacture of vegan products that need to be considered in order to reduce the vegan industry's carbon footprint. Through looking at the case study presented by Choi and Lee, we learned that there has been a climb in the demand for vegan products and materials in recent years. This chapter demonstrated that through open discussion and education, the improvement of the way we produce and consume products is possible— even those that are vegan — for the sake of the Earth.

Some lessons we learned in this chapter:

- The production of vegan goods is beneficial for the environment, but still has room for improvement in manufacturing, farming practices, and transportation.

- According to our recent studies and knowledge, a vegan diet coupled with a vegan lifestyle is one of the best ways you can live in order to reduce your carbon footprint.

- Social media is an avenue for the growth of the vegan diet and lifestyle, as well as inspiration for vegan trends, recipes, clothing items, and discussion of environmental issues caused by animal production.

# CONCLUSION

We have finished our journey together in exploring the endless possibilities of your diet transformation, having investigated the three diets that are central in this guide — the plant-based diet, the vegetarian diet, and the vegan diet. We began by defining the ever-growing plant-based diet, looking at an example of what a plant-based meal would consist of and what researchers and the general public think of this diet. We observed the potential of this diet's food and nutrients, and went into detail in our discussion of the health effects of the plant-based diet. While there are many health benefits of this diet, which is one of the main reasons this diet has become so popular, we also identified the possible health risks that stem from following this diet if not implemented correctly. The health benefits do ultimately outweigh the health risks and issues of this diet because it encourages one to incorporate a variety of plant-based foods that do not pose any risk to our bodies. These specific foods usually do not have additives, preservatives, or harmful substances like most pre-prepared, processed, and packaged foods; due to this factor, we could see that the plant-based diet encourages one to go back to their natural dietary behaviors of our homo-sapien ancestors. This diet is diverse, involving all food groups that are created naturally, sustainably, and ethically — this only improves the well-being of our health and our planet, as less waste and greenhouse gas emissions are produced from the lower production and animal farming demands.

The next topic we investigated was the vegetarian diet. We learned that this diet is more of an umbrella diet, as there exists more specific or sub-diets that fall under the term "vegetarian". This diet is much more diverse and allows its followers more freedom with what can be consumed, allowing animal products like eggs, cheese and even poultry on occasion. This diet has become popular because of the accessibility of it and the extensive amounts of different vegetarian food brands and foods offered. The main rule or restriction for a vegetarian diet is to not eat meat; apart from this rule, one is able to explore different vegetarian food and meal options. You can choose to bake delicious goods that require eggs in the recipe, or you could use a plant-based milk like almond milk instead of cow's milk in the same recipe. The freedom to choose is yours. While vegetarian foods like dairy products still contribute to the carbon footprint of the global population, we learned from the studies we read that the farming of ruminant animals, such as cows and sheep, is one of the main contributing agricultural factors that are harming our planet. Since the vegetarian diet is less restrictive, it can be used as an introduction into receiving the health benefits and environmental changes from reducing consumption of animal products. In our discussions of the health effects and environmental effects of the vegetarian diet, we saw a pattern amongst the people who follow this diet. The positive effects on one's health that were received from consuming a vegetarian diet inspired people to transform their lifestyle more by meditating or exercising. Similarly, we learned that people who are interested in starting the vegetarian diet for environmental reasons became more educated and interested in environmental and animal welfare issues, increasing their dedication to the motivations and causes that made them consider the diet to begin with.

Lastly, we learned about the popular and trendy vegan diet. We defined this diet as the most restrictive out of all three diets — although this diet is not as easy to follow, it does result in a better impact on the environment, as it does not involve any production or demand of animal products. The vegan diet brings about many health benefits, especially if you are transitioning from a typical "western" omnivorous diet to this particular diet of only vegetables, fruits, grains, and legumes. However, you should take a daily supplement of vitamin B-12, as well as additional micronutrients that can be difficult to receive from a vegan diet. While the vegan diet has many significant health benefits, such as lower blood pressure and cholesterol, it also has the most health risks because it excludes two of the major food groups-dairy and animal protein. We learned through analyzing several studies that you should be aware of the specific amounts of macronutrients and micronutrients your body needs; consulting a general practitioner, a dietician or your local pharmacist is a great way to remain informed and supported on your vegan journey. In our discussion on the environmental effects of the vegan diet, we learned that being "vegan" also refers to a specific lifestyle, which transcends the daily foods you consume and refers to all consumer products that do not consist of animal materials or byproducts. Our investigation into the vegan lifestyle and movement revealed the demand and need for more vegan materials, as well as sustainable, biodegradable, recyclable, and cruelty-free products. By demanding for and purchasing vegan, sustainable, and ethical products, "going vegan" will influence the behavior of the marketplace and others around you.

It would be beneficial for your health and for the environment to follow a vegan diet, but it would also be beneficial to purchase ethical and sustainable products packaged in biodegradable or recyclable materials. While you do need to consider your health and nutritional needs, your budget, your cultural routines, and your personal preferences, altering your diet can result in a positive change for your mind, body, and the environment. We have explored the plant-based, vegetarian, and vegan diets in great detail in hopes to inform and inspire. Now, it is up to you to take the first steps in your individual and personal journey. Good luck!

# REFERENCES

Allen, K. E., Gumber, D., & Ostfeld, R. J. (2019). Heart Failure and a Plant-Based Diet. A Case-Report and Literature Review. *Frontiers in Nutrition, 6.* https://doi.org/10.3389/fnut.2019.00082

Bacon, L., & Krpan, D. (2018). (Not) Eating for the environment: The impact of restaurant menu design on vegetarian food choice. *Appetite, 125*, 190–200. https://doi.org/10.1016/j.appet.2018.02.006

Chai, B. C., van der Voort, J. R., Grofelnik, K., Eliasdottir, H. G., Klöss, I., & Perez-Cueto, F. J. A. (2019). Which Diet Has the Least Environmental Impact on Our Planet? A Systematic Review of Vegan, Vegetarian and Omnivorous Diets. *Sustainability, 11*(15), 4110. https://doi.org/10.3390/su11154110

Chen, Z., Zuurmond, M. G., van der Schaft, N., Nano, J., Wijnhoven, H. A. H., Ikram, M. A., Franco, O. H., & Voortman, T. (2018). Plant versus animal based diets and insulin resistance, prediabetes and type 2 diabetes: the Rotterdam Study. *European Journal of Epidemiology, 33*(9), 883–893. https://doi.org/10.1007/s10654-018-0414-8

Choi, Y.-H., & Lee, K.-H. (2021). Ethical Consumers 'Awareness of Vegan Materials: Focused on Fake Fur and Fake Leather. *Sustainability, 13*(1), 436. https://doi.org/10.3390/su13010436

Craig, W. J. (2009). Health effects of vegan diets. *The American Journal of Clinical Nutrition, 89*(5), 1627S1633S. https://doi.org/10.3945/ajcn.2009.26736n

Davey, D., Malone, S., & Egan, B. (2021). Case Study: Transition to a Vegan Diet in an Elite Male Gaelic Football Player. *Sports, 9*(1), 6. https://doi.org/10.3390/sports9010006

Dinu, M., Abbate, R., Gensini, G. F., Casini, A., & Sofi, F. (2016). Vegetarian, vegan diets and multiple health outcomes: A systematic review with meta-analysis of observational studies. *Critical Reviews in Food Science and Nutrition, 57*(17), 3640–3649. https://doi.org/10.1080/10408398.2016.1138447

Eshel, G., Stainier, P., Shepon, A., & Swaminathan, A. (2019). Environmentally Optimal, Nutritionally Sound, Protein and Energy Conserving Plant Based Alternatives to U.S. Meat. *Scientific Reports, 9*(1). https://doi.org/10.1038/s41598-019-46590-1

Fox, Nick, and Katie Ward. "Health, Ethics and Environment: A Qualitative Study of Vegetarian Motivations." *Appetite*, vol. 50, no. 2-3, Mar. 2008, pp. 422–429, 10.1016/j.appet.2007.09.007.

Harvard Health Publishing. (2020, April 15). *Becoming a vegetarian - Harvard Health*. Harvard Health; Harvard Medical School. https://www.health.harvard.edu/staying-healthy/becoming-a-vegetarian

Kahleova, H., Fleeman, R., Hlozkova, A., Holubkov, R., & Barnard, N. D. (2018). A plant-based diet in overweight individuals in a 16-week randomized clinical trial: metabolic benefits of plant protein. *Nutrition & Diabetes, 8*(1). https://doi.org/10.1038/s41387-018-0067-4

Kerschke-Risch, P. (2015). Vegan diet: motives, approach and duration. *Science & Research, 62*(6), 98–103. https://doi.org/10.4455/eu.2015.016

Key, T. J., Appleby, P. N., & Rosell, M. S. (2006). Health effects of vegetarian and vegan diets. *Proceedings of the Nutrition Society, 65*(01), 35–41. https://doi.org/10.1079/pns2005481

Lea, E. J., Crawford, D., & Worsley, A. (2006). Public views of the benefits and barriers to the consumption of a plant-based diet. *European Journal of Clinical Nutrition, 60*(7), 828–837. https://doi.org/10.1038/sj.ejcn.1602387

*Lose It! - Calorie counting made easy.* (2019). Loseit.com. https://www.loseit.com/

Marlow, H. J., Hayes, W. K., Soret, S., Carter, R. L., Schwab, E. R., & Sabaté, J. (2009). Diet and the environment: does what you eat matter? *The American Journal of Clinical Nutrition, 89*(5), 1699S1703S. https://doi.org/10.3945/ajcn.2009.26736z

McCracken, R. D. (1971). Lactase Deficiency: An Example of Dietary Evolution. *Current Anthropology, 12*(4/5), 479–517. https://www.jstor.org/stable/2740932?seq=1

Mock, J., & Schwartz, J. (2019, August 27). What if We All Ate a Bit Less Meat? (Published 2019). *The New York Times.* https://www.nytimes.com/2019/08/21/climate/what-if-we-all-ate-a-bit-less-meat.html#:~:text=So%2C%20according-ing%20to%20a%20study

NHS. (2019). *What should my daily intake of calories be?* NHS. https://www.nhs.uk/common-health-questions/food-and-diet/what-should-my-daily-intake-of-calories-be/

Ostfeld, R. J. (2017). Definition of a plant-based diet and overview of this special issue. *Journal of Geriatric Cardiology : JGC*, *14*(5), 315. https://doi.org/10.11909/j.issn.1671-5411.2017.05.008

Pawlak, R. (2017). Vegetarian Diets in the Prevention and Management of Diabetes and Its Complications. *Diabetes Spectrum*, *30*(2), 82–88. https://doi.org/10.2337/ds16-0057

Pimentel, D., & Pimentel, M. (2003). Sustainability of meat-based and plant-based diets and the environment. *The American Journal of Clinical Nutrition*, *78*(3), 660S663S. https://doi.org/10.1093/ajcn/78.3.660s

Pohjolainen, P., Vinnari, M., & Jokinen, P. (2015). Consumers 'perceived barriers to following a plant-based diet. *British Food Journal*, *117*(3), 1150–1167. https://doi.org/10.1108/bfj-09-2013-0252

Ryan-Harshman, M., & Aldoori, W. (2006). New dietary reference intakes for macronutrients and fibre. *Canadian Family Physician*, *52*(2), 177–179. https://www.ncbi.nlm.nih.gov/pmc/articles/PMC1479724/#:~:text=Dietary%20reference%20intakes%20suggest%20that

Van de Kamp, M. E., & Temme, E. H. M. (2018). Plant-Based Lunch at Work: Effects on Nutrient Intake, Environmental Impact and Tastiness—A Case Study. *Sustainability*, *10*(1), 227. https://doi.org/10.3390/su10010227

Vega, J., Younes, M., & Kuriakose, P. (2008). The Significance of Unexplained Macrocytosis. *Blood*, *112*(11), 3449–3449. https://doi.org/10.1182/blood.v112.11.3449.3449